# MRA Coding Guidelines

# 2018-2019

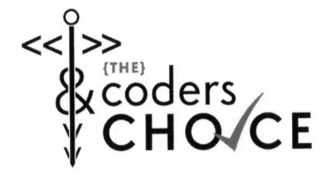

MEDICARE RISK ADJUSTMENT CODING GUIDELINES

# Table of Contents

| | |
|---|---|
| **Introduction** | 2 |
| **Client Profile** | 4 |
| **Substantiation Guide** | 4 |
| **Documentation Requirements** | 4 |
|     Rejecting a Chart | 4 |
|     Patient Information | 5 |
|     Second Patient Identifiers | 5 |
|     Date of Service | 6 |
|     Acceptable Documentation | 6 |
|     Radiology Documentation | 7 |
|     Unacceptable Documentation | 8 |
|     Facility Information | 9 |
|     Skilled Nursing Facilities | 10 |
|     Provider Specialty Type | 10 |
|     Provider Signatures | 12 |
|     Medical Record Documentation Issues | 14 |
|     Abbreviations | 14 |
|     Symbols | 14 |
| **Substantiation** | 15 |
|     Acute vs Chronic | 16 |
|     Medication Lists | 17 |
|     Medications for Substantiation | 17 |
| **General Coding Guidelines** | 18 |
|     Inpatient Place of Service | 18 |
|     Outpatient Place of Service | 19 |
|     History Of | 19 |
|     "With" in ICD-10 | 19 |
|     Other Codes | 19 |
|     Unspecified Codes | 20 |
|     Combination Codes | 20 |
| **Specific Coding Guidelines** | 20 |
|     Lipids | 20 |
|     BMI | 21 |
|     Dialysis Status | 21 |
| **Error** | 21 |
| **Final Signature Page** | 22 |

MEDICARE RISK ADJUSTMENT CODING GUIDELINES

# Client Profile

| | |
|---|---|
| **Project Scope:** | HCC/RxHCC |
| **DOS to be Reviewed:** | 2017/2018 DOS |
| **Estimated Kick-off Date:** | 04/17/2018 |
| **Completion Deadline:** | 3/31/2019 |
| **Focus Area:** | HCC Retrospective – All HCC/RxHCC Only |
| **Reporting Frequency:** | Every DOS |
| **Client Required Audit %:** | 100% first 30 Days, 15% after |
| **Required Quality:** | 95% |
| **Rendering Provider:** | Yes |

## Resources

The following resources have been used in the development of these coding guidelines.

- 2018 ICD-10 CM Official Coding and Reporting Guidelines
- AHA Coding Clinic for ICD-10-CM
- 2008 Risk Adjustment Data Technical Assistance for Medicare Advantage Organizations Participant Guide

# Rejecting a Chart

Prior to coding a chart, the coder must verify that the chart is appropriate for coding.

| Rejection Reason | Definition |
|---|---|
| **Face sheet/Coversheet only** | The chart contains only a face sheet or coversheet and no additional documents. |
| **No Visits within DOS Range** | The entire chart contains DOS outside of the 2017/2018 DOS range. |
| **Comingles-Multiple patients in File** | There is more than one patient records within the chart. |
| **Incorrect or Mismatch DOB** | The DOB does not match. |
| **No Attachment or Illegible Content** | The chart contains no attachment. |
| **Incomplete Notes** | The entire chart contains notes that are not complete (missing pages, missing pieces of the SOAP note). |

MEDICARE RISK ADJUSTMENT CODING GUIDELINES

| Unacceptable POS | The entire chart contains notes that are from an unacceptable place of service, see pages 8-10. |
|---|---|
| Incorrect Patient | The chart belongs to a different patient. |
| Scanning Issue | The chart is not code-able due to a scanning issue. |
| Labs/Imaging Reports only (Excluding Pathology Reports) | The entire chart contains labs/unacceptable radiology reports that are not acceptable documents to code from. |

# Documentation Requirements

## Patient Information

The correct patient name must match the entire medical record

- When the patient's entire name does not match throughout the chart but there is only one patient's information in the chart - reject the chart for incorrect patient.
- When the patient's first name does not match but is a common nickname the - chart should be coded.
- When the patient's name matches on some notes and there is another patient's information in the chart - reject the chart for multiple patients.
- When there is a patient pull list in the chart - reject the chart for multiple patients.
- When there are minor spelling errors either in the first name or last name but the DOB matches - chart should be coded.
- When the last name is inconsistent throughout the chart - reject the chart for multiple patients.

## Second Patient Identifiers

Each DOS must have the correct patient name and an additional second patient identifier documented.

| The second patient identifier can be any one of the following: ||
|---|---|
| Any Geographical subdivision smaller than a state. This can include street address, city, county precinct, zip code or their equivalent geocodes. ||
| Date of Birth | SSN or last 4 digits of the SSN |
| Medical Record Number (MRN) | Health Plan Beneficiary Number |
| Account Number | Certificate/License Number |
| Vehicle Identifiers and Serial numbers, including license plate number | Device identifiers and serial numbers |
| Web Universal Resource Locators (URLs) | Internet Protocol (IP) address numbers |
| Biometric Identifiers, including finger and voice prints | Phone number or fax number |

## MEDICARE RISK ADJUSTMENT CODING GUIDELINES

| Electronic mail address (email) | Full Face photographic images and any comparable images |
|---|---|
| Medicare Number/HICN | |

- When a medical record is missing the second patient identifier the record will still be coded and the 'Missing Second Patient Identifier' error comment will be appended to each diagnosis from that DOS.
- When the name matches, but the DOB does not match for the entire record, reject the chart for incorrect DOB.
- When the name matches and some DOS have a matching DOB and other do not, code only the DOS with the correct DOB.

## Date of Service

A clear date of service must be present at least once on the document.
- Records without a clear date of service will not be coded.
- A vital signs date can be used as the date of service only when it is not contracted somewhere else in the note.
- Signature dates cannot be used as the date of service.
- Discharge summaries will be coded using the discharge date.
- Consultation notes will be coded using the consult date.
- Pathology reports will be coded using the collection date.
- Letters can be coded when they meet the acceptable documentation requirements and there is either a specific DOS note or the date of the letter should be used when the verbiage 'I have seen 'the patient' today'.

## Acceptable Documentation

Acceptable records to capture diagnosis codes from must involve a face-to-face visit with the patient from an acceptable physician specialty
- Evidence of a face-to-face visit includes:
- Patient seen today ...
- Patient presents today ...
- Objective data including examinations, lab results, vital signs, etc.
- Discussed, reviewed, explained, etc.

## MEDICARE RISK ADJUSTMENT CODING GUIDELINES

| Acceptable records must contain all elements of a SOAP note. | |
|---|---|
| Subjective | How the patient describes their problem or illness |
| Objective | Data obtained from examinations, lab results, vital signs, etc. |
| Assessment | List of the patient's current condition and status of all chronic conditions. How the objective data relate to the patient's acute problem. |
| Plan | Next steps in diagnosing problem further, prescriptions, consultation referrals, patient education, and recommended time to return for follow-up. |

**Acceptable Documents to code from include:**
- Inpatient History and Physical (H&P)
- Consultations (Inpatient and Outpatient)
- Emergency Department (ED) Visits
- Discharge Summary (with a discharge date)
- Operation Reports
- Outpatient Progress Notes
- Health Risk Assessment (HRA) forms-with evidence of a face-to-face visit
- Hospital day to day visits
- Lab results and diagnostic radiology results can be coded when they are embedded into a face-to-face visit
- Summaries (Clinical, Patient, Visit) can be coded if the summary has all elements of a SOAP notes
- Pathology Report-Collection date must be used as the DOS
  - Examples of pathology reports
  - Pathology report from a tissue biopsy (e.g., lung biopsy, breast biopsy, etc.)
  - Cell block report
  - Cytopathology report of fluids, brushings
  - Papanicolaou (PAP) smear report
  - Chromosome analysis

## Radiology Documentation

- Radiological procedures that are summarized by the provider and/or discussed with the patient during that visit are acceptable to abstract from. There must be some type of action plan or MEAT to support the diagnosis abstracted.
- If there is a radiological report that is embedded in the note and is not summarized by the provider or reviewed with the patient during the visit it is not acceptable.

Certain minimally invasive procedures that do not involve a face-to-face visit are allowed for risk adjustment when they meet the below requirements.

- The following radiology procedures can be coded when a CMS approved provider provides interpretation.

## MEDICARE RISK ADJUSTMENT CODING GUIDELINES

> If the reason for the test is to rule out a diagnosis, do not code the diagnosis if the exam is normal or does not indicate the rule out diagnosis.

**Acceptable radiology procedures include:**
- Cardiology and Vascular
    - Echocardiogram (including Doppler, Duplex, Color flow of the heart vessels)
    - Electrocardiogram (EKG)-Stress test, Cardiac catheterization
    - Myocardial perfusion and other nuclear medicine imaging of the heart
    - Pacemaker analysis (non-telephonic)
    - Vascular Doppler Study interpretation - not performed by Diagnostic Radiologists
    - Percutaneous transluminal coronary angiography (PTCA)
- Interventional Radiology
    - Catheter angiography - Coronary Computed tomography angiography (CTA)
    - Endoscopic retrograde cholangiopancreatography (ERCP)
    - Embolization procedures
    - Extracorporeal shock wave lithotripsy (ESWL)
    - Magnetic resonance arteriogram (MRA)
    - Fluoroscopic Guidance
    - Genitourinary vascular flow imaging (nuclear medicine)
    - Radiofrequency ablation
    - Radiation Therapy-Ultrasound Guidance
- Neurology
    - Electroencephalography (EEG)
    - Electromyography (EMG)
    - Nerve Conduction Studies
    - Nuclear Medicine Brain Imaging
    - Sleep Studies (Polysomnography)
- Pulmonology
    - Pulmonary Function Tests (PFT)
    - Pulmonary perfusion and ventilation imaging

## Unacceptable Documentation

Unacceptable notes to code from include:
- Ambulance
- Claims data
- Laboratory Services
- Superbills
- Supplies

## MEDICARE RISK ADJUSTMENT CODING GUIDELINES

- Diagnostic Radiology Services
- Coumadin Clinic Notes when the patient is only seen by the RN
- Nursing Visit Notes
- Case Manager Notes
- Prosthetics
- Respite care facilities
- Stand-alone problem lists
- Durable medical equipment
- Hospice and home health care
- Intermediate care facility notes

## Facility Information

| MRA Covered Hospital Inpatient Facilities | **MRA Non-Covered Hospital Inpatient Facilities** |
|---|---|
| Short-term (general and specialty) Hospitals | Skilled Nursing Facilities (SNF) |
| Religious Non-Medical Health Care Institutions | Hospital Inpatient Swing Bed Components |
| Long-term Hospitals | Intermediate Care Facilities |
| Rehabilitation Hospitals | Respite Care |
| Children's Hospitals | Hospice |
| Psychiatric Hospitals | |
| Medical Assistance Facilities/Critical Access Hospitals | |

*Not an All-Inclusive list

| MRA Covered Hospital Outpatient Facilities | **MRA Non-Covered Hospital Outpatient Facilities** |
|---|---|
| Short-term (general and specialty) Hospitals | Free-standing Ambulatory Surgical Centers (ASCs) |
| Medical Assistance Facilities/Critical Access Hospitals | Home Health Care |
| Community Mental Health Centers | Free-standing Renal Dialysis Facilities Non-Covered Services |
| Federally Qualified Health Centers | Laboratory Services |
| Religious Non-Medical Health Care Institutions | Ambulance |
| Long-term Hospitals | Durable Medical Equipment |
| Rehabilitation Hospitals | Prosthetics |
| Children's Hospitals | Orthotics |
| Psychiatric Hospitals | Supplies |
| Rural Health Clinic (Free-standing and Provider Based) | Radiology Services |

*Not an All-Inclusive list

| Acceptable Place of Service | |
|---|---|
| Assisted Living Facility | Military Treatment Facility |
| Birthing Center | Mobile Unit |
| Community Mental Health Center | Nonresidential Substance Abuse Treatment Facility |

MEDICARE RISK ADJUSTMENT CODING GUIDELINES

| | |
|---|---|
| Comprehensive Inpatient Rehabilitation Facility | Office |
| Comprehensive Outpatient Rehabilitation Facility | Outpatient Hospital |
| Emergency Room – Hospital | Psychiatric Facility Partial Hospitalization |
| End-Stage Renal Disease Treatment Facility | Psychiatric Residential Treatment Center |
| Federal Qualified Health Center | Public Health Center |
| Group Home | Residential Substance Abuse Treatment Facility |
| Home | Rural Health Clinic |
| Independent Clinic | Temporary Lodging |
| Indian Health Service Freestanding Facility | Tribal 638 Freestanding Facility |
| Indian Health Service Provider-Based Facility | Tribal 638 Provider-Based Facility |
| Inpatient Hospital | Urgent Care |
| Inpatient Psychiatric Facility | Walk-in Retail Health Clinic |
| Intermediate Care Facility/Mentally Retarded | |

| **Unacceptable Place of Service** | |
|---|---|
| Ambulance | Mass Immunization Center |
| Ambulance air or water | Nursing Facility* |
| Ambulatory Surgical Center | Other Place of Service |
| Custodial Care Facility | Pharmacy |
| Description | Prison-Correctional Facility |
| Homeless Shelter | School |
| Hospice | Skilled Nursing Facility* |
| Independent Laboratory | |

## Skilled Nursing Facilities

- Although Skilled Nursing Facilities are not an acceptable place of service, when the following are present within the medical record documentation, the coder should capture codes from a Skilled Nursing Facility record.
- The provider's encounter must have been a face-to-face with the beneficiary
- The clinical provider rendering the services must be an acceptable physician specialty for risk adjustment
- The medical record must clearly document the provider's signature and credentials
- The beneficiary must be identified as a long-term institutional resident.

## Correct Provider Specialty Type

| CMS identifies a list of approved physician specialty types for CMS-HCC risk adjustment coding. This list includes providers such as: | |
|---|---|
| Medical Doctor (MD) | Certified Nurse Midwives (CNM) |
| Doctor of Osteopathic Medicine (DO) | Certified Registered Nurse Anesthetist (CRNA) |

# MEDICARE RISK ADJUSTMENT CODING GUIDELINES

| Advanced Practice Registered Nurse (APRN/APN) | Clinical Nurse Specialists (CNS) |
|---|---|
| Nurse Practitioner (NP) | Advanced Registered Nurse Practitioner (ARNP) |
| Acute Care Nurse Practitioner (ACNP) | Adult Nurse Practitioner (ANP) |
| Physician's Assistant (PA) | Advanced Oncology Certified Nurse Practitioner (AOCNP) |
| Physical Therapist (PT) | Licensed Clinical Social Worker (LCSW) |
| Registered Nurse (RN)-dictating as a scribe for MD | Chiropractor (DC) |

## Acceptable Provider Specialty Type

Documents from an unacceptable physician specialty will not be used.

### Acceptable Medicare Advantage Physician Specialty Types for 2018 Payment Year (2017 DOS)

| Code | Specialty | Code | Specialty | Code | Specialty |
|---|---|---|---|---|---|
| 79 | Addiction Medicine | C7 | Advanced Heart Failure and Transplant Cardiology | 3 | Allergy/ Immunology |
| 5 | Anesthesiology | 64* | Audiologist | 21 | Cardiac Electrophysiology |
| 78 | Cardiac Surgery | 6 | Cardiology | 89* | Certified Clinical Nurse Specialist |
| 42 | Certified Nurse Midwife | 43 | Certified Registered Nurse Anesthetist | 35 | Chiropractic |
| 68 | Clinical Psychologist | 28 | Colorectal Surgery (formerly Proctology) | 81 | Critical care (intensivists) |
| C5 | Dentist | 7 | Dermatology | 93 | Emergency Medicine |
| 46* | Endocrinology | 8 | Family Practice | 10 | Gastroenterology |
| 1 | General Practice | 2 | General Surgery | 38 | Geriatric Medicine |
| 27 | Geriatric Psychiatry | 98 | Gynecologist/ Oncologist | 40 | Hand Surgery |
| 82 | Hematology | 83 | Hematology/ Oncology | C9 | Hematopoietic Cell Transplantation and Cellular Therapy |
| 17 | Hospice and Palliative Care | C6 | Hospitalist | 44 | Infectious Disease |
| 11 | Internal Medicine | C3 | Interventional Radiology | 9 | Interventional Pain Management (IPM) |
| 94 | Interventional Radiology | 80 | Licensed Clinical Social Worker | 85 | Maxillofacial Surgery |
| 90 | Medical Oncology | C8 | Medical Toxicology | 39 | Nephrology |
| 13 | Neurology | 86 | Neuropsychiatry | 14 | Neurosurgery |
| 36 | Nuclear Medicine | 50* | Nurse Practitioner | 16 | Obstetrics/ Gynecology |
| 67 | Occupational Therapist | 18 | Ophthalmology | 41 | Optometry |
| 19 | Oral Surgery (dentists only) | 20 | Orthopedic Surgery | 12 | Osteopathic Manipulative medicine |
| 4 | Otolaryngology | 72* | Pain Management | 22 | Pathology |
| 37 | Pediatric medicine | 76* | Peripheral Vascular Disease | 25 | Physical Medicine and Rehabilitation |

MEDICARE RISK ADJUSTMENT CODING GUIDELINES

| 65 | Physical Therapist | 97* | Physician Assistant | 24 | Plastic and Reconstructive Surgery |
|---|---|---|---|---|---|
| 48* | Podiatry | 84 | Preventative Medicine | 26 | Psychiatry |
| 62* | Psychologist | 29 | Pulmonary Disease | 92 | Radiation Oncology |
| 66 | Rheumatology | C0 | Sleep Medicine | 15 | Speech Language Pathologist |
| 23 | Sports Medicine | 91 | Surgical Oncology | 33* | Thoracic Surgery |
| 99 | Unknown Physician Specialty | 34 | Urology | 77 | Vascular Surgery |

## Additional Provider Specialty Type Guidance

- Medical Assistants (MA, RMA, CMA) are unacceptable provider specialties.
- Nurses (RN, LPN, CNA) are also unacceptable provider specialties.
- Licensed professional counselors (LPC) are not an acceptable provider specialty. Do not assume this is a psychologist or LCSW.
- Licensed Professional Counselor is an unacceptable provider specialties
- Licensed Mental Health Counselor is an unacceptable provider specialty

- PhD – Doctor of Philosophy is not an acceptable credential
- Resident, Post Graduate Medical Students (PG-1, PGY-2) and Hospitalist are acceptable provider specialties.

## Provider Signatures

### Handwritten Signatures
- Handwritten signatures or handwritten initials including provider credentials are acceptable.
- Handwritten signatures do not have to be legible, but you do have to reasonably determine that the signing provider is a valid CMS provider.
- Provider credentials can be found anywhere on the document.
- When a provider name is listed but no provider credentials are found, the note should be coded and the 'No Valid Provider Signature' error comment appended to each diagnosis from that DOS.
- Handwritten signatures do not require a signature date.
- Notes that do not have a provider name will not be coded.
- **Example**:
    - Full name: John M. Smith, MD
    - Initials: JMS, MD

### Electronic Signatures

# MEDICARE RISK ADJUSTMENT CODING GUIDELINES

- Electronic signatures should include three required components:
    1. Electronic verbiage-indicating it is a signature or an authentication (see table below).
    2. Provider name-can be located anywhere on the document
    3. Valid CMS credential-can be located anywhere on the document
- Electronic signatures must be signed within 180 days of the DOS. If the signature date is after the 180 days the note will still be coded and the **'No Valid Provider Signature'** error comment added to each diagnosis from that DOS.
- Notes that do not have a provider name will not be coded.
- When a provider name is listed but no provider credentials are found or the note does not have the proper electronic verbiage, the note should be coded and the 'No Valid Provider Signature' error comment appended to each diagnosis from that DOS.

| Examples of Acceptable EMR Authentication Statements | | |
|---|---|---|
| Accepted by | Digitized signature | Sealed by |
| Acknowledged by | Electronically approved by | Signature Derived from Controlled Access Password |
| Approved by | Electronically authored by | Signature on file (with typed name) |
| Authenticated by | Electronically signed by | Signed |
| Authored by | Entered by | Signed by |
| Authorized by | Entered data sealed by | Signed before import by |
| Charted by | Finalized by | Supervised by |
| Closed by | Generated by | This is an electronically verified report by |
| Completed by | Performed by | Validated by |
| Confirmed by | Read by | Verified by |
| Digital Signature | Released by | Written by |
|  | Reviewed by | Status Pending – When Accompanied with a complete signature |

**Examples of Unacceptable EMR Authentication Statements**
- Notes with the below authentications will still be coded when provider name is present, using the 'No Valid Provider Signature' error comment on each diagnosis from that DOS.
    - Administratively signed
    - Dictated but not read
    - Dictated but no signed
    - Electronically signed by agent of provider
    - Filled by
    - Signature on file

## MEDICARE RISK ADJUSTMENT CODING GUIDELINES

- Signed but not read

## Medical Record Documentation Issues

- Missing Pages
  - If all elements of a SOAP note are present, and documentation meets all other documentation requirements
- Distorted or Poorly Scanned Images
  - Code from legible pages
- Pages or Images cut off
  - Code from legible pages
- Addendums/Amendments
  - In order to code from an addendum, the following must apply:
    - The addendum must be based on an observation of the patient on the date of service.
    - Signed by the treating provider of the original encounter
    - Addendums should be dated within 90 days of the encounter

## Abbreviations

- Several abbreviations have more than one meaning
- Evaluate the abbreviation within the context of the full medical record
- If more than one condition is present in the record that could apply to the abbreviation, you must have MEAT to support the code selection.
  - **Example 1**: PVD in an Ophthalmologist chart does not mean peripheral vascular disease, but instead means posterior vitreous detachment
  - **Example 2**: RA could mean rheumatoid arthritis OR reactive arthritis
  - **Example 3**: MI could mean myocardial infarction OR mental illness OR mitral insufficiency

## Symbols

| | Symbols |
|---|---|
| ? | Do not code when used as bullet points in a list |
| / | Do not assume a link between the conditions or diagnosis, consider the "/" to read as "and" |
| ↑ | Do not code as "increase" in front of a condition |
| ↓ | Do not code as "decrease" in front of a condition |
| s̄ | Means without |

MEDICARE RISK ADJUSTMENT CODING GUIDELINES

| C | Means with |
|---|---|

# Substantiation

## Substantiation Guide

> Coding a condition depends on where it is found in the chart note and whether or not it has MEAT. Please see the below table for further information.

|  | Chronic |
|---|---|
| CC | Y w/MEAT |
| HPI | Y |
| ROS | Y w/MEAT |
| PMH | Y |
| PL | Y w/MEAT |
| PE | Yes |
| Assessment | Yes |
| Plan | Yes |
| Med List | Insulin Only |

| **Substantiation Guide Exceptions** | |
|---|---|
| Require MEAT regardless of location | Can be captured from any portion of the note regardless if MEAT is present |
| DVT, PE, Cancers NOT identified as Chronic, MI, CVA and AAA, Dialysis Status and/or -Ostomy | Old MI, Amputation Status and Transplant Status, |

> Depending on where the condition is found in the chart note it may need substantiation confirming the condition is still present. The concept of substantiation is also expressed through the acronym MEAT. Below are examples of substantiation, this is not an all-inclusive list.

| MEAT (only 1 is required) | |
|---|---|
| Monitor | Noting signs or symptoms of the disease that are present |
| | Noting disease regression or progression |
| | Commonly found in HPI, ROS and/or physical exam |
| Evaluate | Reviewing lab, pathology, radiology results |
| | Diagnostic testing that is performed during the same calendar year as the diagnoses can be considered support for the condition |
| | Discussion of progress towards health goal |
| | Findings in the physical exam |
| Assess/ Address | The condition may be addressed in a narrative HPI by the provider |
| | The condition may be assessed in the physical exam |
| | Diagnostic test/labs ordered. Orders do not need to be directly correlated to the condition |
| | Follow up is scheduled |
| Treat | Physical or occupational therapy |

MEDICARE RISK ADJUSTMENT CODING GUIDELINES

| | |
|---|---|
| Patient refusal of treatment for a condition | |
| Referral to a specialist | |
| Medication (see medication section of guidelines) | |

# Acute vs. Chronic

## Acute Conditions

> Acute conditions are severe and sudden in onset. This could describe anything from a broken bone to an asthma attack.

| | Acute |
|---|---|
| CC | Y w/MEAT |
| HPI | Y w/MEAT |
| ROS | Y w/MEAT |
| PMH | Y w/MEAT |
| PL | Y w/MEAT |
| PE | Y w/MEAT |
| Assessment | Y w/MEAT |
| Plan | Y w/MEAT |

**Acute Codes - When MEAT is present, capture the code

**Acute Codes - When MEAT is not present, do not code

## Chronic Conditions

> A chronic condition is a long-developing syndrome, such as osteoporosis or asthma.

| | Chronic |
|---|---|
| CC | Y w/MEAT |
| HPI | Y |
| ROS | Y w/MEAT |
| PMH | Y |
| PL | Y w/MEAT |
| PE | Yes |
| Assessment | Yes |
| Plan | Yes |

*See exceptions table

**When MEAT is present, capture the code

**When MEAT is required for capturing a chronic conditions based on the guide to the left, and no MEAT is found, capture the chronic condition and append the **No Supporting Documentation** error comment

# Medication Lists

## Long Term Use Medications

## MEDICARE RISK ADJUSTMENT CODING GUIDELINES

- The only HCC/Rx HCC captured from the medication list is for long term use of insulin. In an out-patient setting, it is not necessary to see diabetes documented in the chart to capture this status code, but "long term use" must be validated.
- If Type I Diabetes and insulin are documented on the document, capture both codes.
- If DM Type I is documented on the note and no insulin is documented then the correct code would be DM unspecified, E11.9, and the coder would not capture Z79.4 since there is no insulin documented in the note.
- Code Z79.4, should not be assigned if the insulin is given temporarily (i.e. sliding scale insulin) to bring a patient's type II diabetes under control. (2017 Official Coding Guideline I.C.4.a.3

## Medications used for support

- Prescription (RX) are acceptable substantiation
- Over the Counter (OTC) medications can be used only when they are called out for the conditions.
    - **Example**: Patient is taking aspirin for CAD
- Medications found in a current medication list that is part of the face to face encounter are to be used as substantiation for the condition. There does not need to be an indication that medication was reviewed or changed on that date of service.
- Medications found in other parts of the progress note such as the Plan can be used for substantiation.
- Use the following guidelines if the medication can be used for numerous conditions:
    - If only one condition is present and one acceptable medication is present, use the medication as substantiation.
    - If multiple conditions are present and there is only one acceptable medication present, the rendering provider must directly correlate the condition to the medication to be used as substantiation for an acute or chronic condition in order for the condition to be captured. With the exception of Lipid codes (see page 20)

        - **Acute** - If the condition is an acute condition and there is no correlation between the condition and the medication the code is not to be captured.

        - **Chronic** - If the condition is a chronic condition and there is no correlation, the code is to be captured and flagged with the error comment No supporting documentation. Lipids are an exception, see below

        - **Lipids** - One medication can be used to substantiate multiple lipid conditions located in the same DOS (see page 20). If there is an acute condition and a lipid condition(s) present and the same medication could treat both the acute and the lipid condition(s), but the rendering provider has not made the correlation, the acute condition is not coded, and the lipid condition(s) is coded with the error comment **No supporting documentation**.

MEDICARE RISK ADJUSTMENT CODING GUIDELINES

- **Example 1**: Cymbalta is on the medication list and depression is documented with no neurological diagnoses noted (or any other condition that Cymbalta can be prescribed for), then Cymbalta can be used as a validator for depression.

- **Example 2**: If Cymbalta is on the medication list and depression and neuropathy is noted and the rendering provider has not made a correlation, then Cymbalta cannot be used to validate depression or neuropathy. In this case (depression is considered acute/chronic) neuropathy is the only condition that would be coded with the error comment No Supporting Documentation.

> Do not assume conditions from the presence of a medication.

# General Coding Guidelines

> Follow all ICD-10 Guidelines except when specified differently in the chapter specific guidelines
> Numeric diagnosis code without a description cannot be abstracted.
> All diagnoses should be coded to the highest level of specificity based on the provider's documentation. Some conditions are described by more than one term depending on the clinical presentation and medical terminology practices of the physician. (2017 Official Coding Guideline I.B.18)
> Some single diagnoses require more than one code to accurately capture the condition. Follow all instructional notes at the block, category, sub-category, and code levels in the tabular. (2017 Official Coding Guideline I.B.7).
> Conditions that are integral to each other should not be coded separately. (2017 Official Coding Guideline I.B.5.)
  - **Example**: Depression is an integral component of bipolar disorder and therefore depression should not be coded separately.
> Conditions that are described in one combination code, should not be coded separately unless instructional notes require otherwise. (2017 Official Coding Guideline I.B.9)
  - **Example 1**: F10.24 is assigned to alcohol dependence with mood disorder. Only one code is needed to capture both conditions.
  - **Example 2**: E11.22 is assigned to DM type 2 with CKD. Although this is a combination code, instructional notes require an additional code to be used for the stage of the CKD.
> All captured codes must be supported as present during that visit by the documentation of the visit. The provider's statement that a patient has a particular condition is sufficient with or without evidence of the clinical criteria used by the provider to establish the diagnosis (2017 Official Guideline I.A.19.). Refer to Chart Note Components on page 2 of this document for specific clarification.

## Inpatient Place of Service

## MEDICARE RISK ADJUSTMENT CODING GUIDELINES

- When a medical record is part of an inpatient stay such as short-term, acute, long-term care and psychiatric hospitals if the diagnosis documented at the time of discharge is qualified as "probable", "suspected", "likely", "questionable", "possible", or "still to be ruled out", code the condition as if it existed or was established. (2017 Official Coding Guideline III.C.)
- If at the time of discharge, the provider is stating a comparative/contrasting diagnosis, code the condition(s) as if it existed or was established. (Coding Clinic, 2nd Qtr., 2016)
- Example: Discharge summary diagnosis-TIA vs. CVA

## Outpatient Place of Service

- Do not capture unconfirmed diagnosis codes such as "probable fracture", "suspected MI", "questionable CVA", "likely pulmonary embolism". The following synonyms are also considered unconfirmed: "rule out", "consistent with", "working", "compatible with", "indicative of", "suggestive of" and "comparable with". Rather, the condition(s) shall be coded to the highest degree of certainty known for that encounter/visit such as signs and symptoms, abnormal test results or other reason(s) for the face-to-face visit. (2017 Official Coding Guideline IV. H.) (Coding Clinic, 1st Qtr., 2014)
- When the provider documents "evidence of" a particular condition, it is not considered an uncertain diagnosis and should be appropriately coded..." (Coding Clinic, 3rd Qtr., 2009 and Coding Clinic, 1st Qtr., 2014)

## "History Of"

- When a diagnosis is stated as "history of" but we have substantiation that it is an active/current condition on that date of service, we would code the condition as current. (2017 Official Coding Guideline I.C.21.c.4.)
- A true "history of" diagnosis means that the patient no longer has the condition nor is receiving treatment for that condition.
- Clear documentation is essential to make the appropriate determination. "History of" codes may be used as secondary codes if the historical condition has an impact on current care or influences treatment. If the provider documents a current condition as a "history of", and it is on the HCC list as a chronic condition, the coder may submit the code as a current chronic condition.

## "With" in ICD-10

- The word "with" should be interpreted to mean "associated with" or "due to" when it appears in a code title. The classification presumes a causal relationship between the two conditions linked by these terms. These conditions should be coded as related even in the absence of provider documentation explicitly linking them, unless the documentation clearly states the conditions are unrelated. For conditions not specifically linked by these relational terms in the classification, provider documentation must link the conditions in order to code them as related.

## "Other" Codes

- Codes titled "other" or "other specified" are for use when the information in the medical record provides detail for which a specific code does not exist. Alphabetic index entries with

# MEDICARE RISK ADJUSTMENT CODING GUIDELINES

NEC in the line designate "other" codes in the tabular list. These alphabetic index entries represent specific disease entities for which no specific code exists, so the term is included within an "other" code. In cases where a provider has documented as "other specified", detail in the record must exist classifying what the specified condition is. In cases where there is not further specificity within the note regarding the condition, the unspecified code should be selected.

| Documentation States: | Correct Code Captured: |
|---|---|
| Other hyperlipidemia | E78.4, other hyperlipidemia |
| Other hypothyroidism | E03.8, other specified hypothyroidism |
| Other peripheral vascular disease | I73.89, other specified peripheral vascular diseases |

## Unspecified Codes

> Not otherwise specified (NOS): Means "unspecified." Unspecified codes are for use when the documentation does not provide additional information to assign a more specific code. Unspecified codes should be used when a condition is indexed but further specificity from the provider cannot be found within the date of service. In most cases where you cannot index a condition, it would not be appropriate to assign an unspecified code to the condition.
>> • Example: Provider has documented hyperlipidemia in the Assessment portion of the note. No further specification is found within the same note, Capture E78.5 – Unspecified Hyperlipidemia.

## Combination Codes

> When a combination code is present for two conditions, based on the substantiation guide, if one or both conditions are pulled from a portion of the note that requires substantiation, both conditions should be substantiated in order to capture the combination code.

> Conditions that are described in one combination code, should not be coded separately unless instructional notes require otherwise. (2017 Official Coding Guideline I.B.9)
>> • **Example 1**: F10.24 is assigned to alcohol dependence with mood disorder. Only one code is needed to capture both conditions.
>> • **Example 2**: E11.22 is assigned to DM type 2 with CKD. Although this is a combination code, instructional notes require an additional code to be used for the stage of the CKD.

# Specific Coding Guidelines

## Lipids

> Each lipid diagnosis stands alone, so you can capture multiple lipid codes in the same DOS
> One medication can be used to substantiate multiple lipid codes on the same DOS
> **Example**: E78.2, E78.00 and E78.5 - Multiple lipid diagnosis are all seen in the same DOS, substantiation is present, each unique code should be captured using the one medication. If

substantiation is not present each unique lipid diagnosis is still captured with the error comment **No supporting documentation.**

## BMI

- If the BMI is documented at or above 40.0, capture the appropriate ICD-10 code (Z68.41 through Z68.45). The BMI can be documented by nurses or other clinic staff and still be coded. (AHA Coding Clinic 2Q 2010 – BMI)
- If the BMI is 40+, but no mention of morbid obesity, you cannot code morbid obesity but you can capture the status code for the BMI. Do NOT capture the diagnosis of "morbid obesity" based solely on the BMI. The provider's documentation must state "morbid obesity". (AHA Coding Clinic 4Q 2008 - Assigning Body Mass Index (BMI) Codes).
- The diagnosis of morbid obesity can be coded without a BMI noted.
- If the BMI is less than 40 and morbid obesity is diagnosed look for additional MEAT to support the condition.

## Dialysis Status

- If the documentation states presence of AV fistula, do not make any assumptions as to the purpose of the fistula, such as "for dialysis". Unless there is clear documentation that the patient is on dialysis, you would not code Z99.2 (AHA Coding Clinic 2Q 2013 - CKD Stage IV with Plans for Starting Dialysis)
- There are two kinds of Peritoneal Dialysis
    - Continuous Ambulatory Peritoneal Dialysis (CAPD)
    - Automated Peritoneal Dialysis (APD)

# Error Comments

The following flags are to be used in the project when applicable:

| Error Comments | Error Comment Description | Chart Level | Code Level |
| --- | --- | --- | --- |
| Missing Second Patient Identifier | When second patient is not found on date of service | | X |
| No Valid Provider Signature | When a required portion of the signature is missing | | X |
| No Supporting Documentation | When MEAT is not present in an area of the note requiring MEAT | | X |
| No HCC Codes | If no HCC codes are found in the entire record | X | |
| No DOS Found | When no acceptable Date of Service is found in Chart | X | |

## Common Medications and Conditions Treated

| Drug | Primary Condition Treated | Other Conditions Treated | Drug Class |
|---|---|---|---|
| Adderall® | ADHD | Narcolepsy | CNS Stimulants |
| Amphetamine | ADHD | Narcolepsy | CNS Stimulants |
| Atomoxetine | ADHD | | CNS Stimulants |
| Concerta® | ADHD | | CNS Stimulants |
| Dexmethylphenidate | ADHD | | CNS Stimulants |
| Focalin® | ADHD | | CNS Stimulants |
| Lisdexamfetamine | ADHD | | CNS Stimulants |
| Methylphenidate | ADHD | | CNS Stimulants |
| Strattera® | ADHD | | CNS Stimulants |
| Vyvanse® | ADHD | | CNS Stimulants |
| Cetirizine | Allergies | | Antihistamines |
| Claritin® | Allergies | | Antihistamines |
| Loratadine | Allergies | | Antihistamines |
| Mometasone | Allergies | | Inhaled Corticosteroid |
| Nasonex® | Allergies | | Nasal Steroid |
| Zyrtec® | Allergies | | Antihistamines |
| Olopatadine | Allergies | | Antihistamines |
| Patanol® | Allergies | | Antihistamines |
| Phenergan® | Allergies | | Antihistamines |
| Promethazine | Allergies | | Antihistamines |
| Flonase® | Allergies - | | Nasal Steroid |
| Fluticasone | Allergies - | | Inhaled Corticosteroid |
| Memantine | Alzheimers | | Misc CNS Agents |
| Namenda® | Alzheimers | | Misc CNS Agents |
| NitroStat® SL | Angina | | Vasodilators |
| Dolophine® | Anti-addictive | | Narcotic Analgesics |
| Methadone | Anti-addictive | | Narcotic Analgesics |
| Alprazolam | Anti-Anxiety | | Benzodiazepines |
| Ativan® | Anti-Anxiety | | Benzodiazepines |
| Buspar® | Anti-anxiety | | Misc Anxiolytics, sedatives and hypnotics |
| Buspirone | Anti-anxiety | | Misc Anxiolytics, sedatives and hypnotics |
| Clonazepam | Anti-Anxiety | | Benzodiazepines |
| Diazepam | Anti-Anxiety | | Benzodiazepines |
| Klonopin® | Anti-Anxiety | | Benzodiazepines |
| Lorazepam | Anti-Anxiety | | Benzodiazepines |
| Valium® | Anti-Anxiety | Muscle Spasms | Benzodiazepines |
| Xanax® | Anti-Anxiety | | Benzodiazepines |
| Advair® | Asthma | COPD | Bronchodilator |
| Albuterol | Asthma | COPD | Bronchodilator |
| Budesonide + Form | Asthma | COPD | Inhaled Corticosteroid |
| Fluticasone + Salme | Asthma | COPD | Inhaled Corticosteroid |
| Montelukast | Asthma | | Leukotriene Modifiers |
| Singulair® | Asthma | | Leukotriene Modifiers |
| Symbicort® | Asthma | COPD | Inhaled Corticosteroid |
| Levalbuterol | Asthma | | Bronchodilator |
| Xopenex® | Asthma | | Bronchodilator |
| ProAir® HFA | Asthma Inhaler | | Bronchodilator |
| Amoxicillin + Clavul | Bacteria Infection | | Anti-biotic |
| Augmentin® | Bacteria Infection | | Anti-biotic |
| Avodart® | Benign Prostatic Hyperplasia | | 5-alpha-reductase Inhibitors |
| Dutasteride | Benign Prostatic Hyperplasia | | 5-alpha-reductase Inhibitors |
| Finasteride | Benign Prostatic Hyperplasia | | 5-alpha-reductase Inhibitors |
| Hytrin® | Benign Prostatic Hyperplasia | | Antiadrenergic Agents |
| Proscar® | Benign Prostatic Hyperplasia | | 5-alpha-reductase Inhibitors |
| Terazosin | Benign Prostatic Hyperplasia | | Antiadrenergic Agents |
| Clopidogrel | Blood Clots | | Anti-Platelet |
| Plavix® | Blood Clots | | Anti-Platelet |
| Coumadin® | Blood Clots | | Anti-Coagulant |
| Rivaroxaban | Blood Clots | | Anti-Coagulant |

## Common Medications and Conditions Treated

| Drug | Primary Condition Treated | Other Conditions Treated | Drug Class |
|---|---|---|---|
| Warfarin | Blood Clots | | Anti-Coagulant |
| Xarelto® | Blood Clots | | Anti-Coagulant |
| Dabigatran | Blood Thinner | | Anti-coagulant |
| Nifedipine | Calc. Chan. Blocker | | Calcium Channel Blocker |
| Procardia® | Calc. Chan. Blocker | | Calcium Channel Blocker |
| Verapamil | Calc. Chan. Blocker | | Calcium Channel Blocker |
| Verelan® | Calc. Chan. Blocker | | Calcium Channel Blocker |
| Amlodipine | Calc. Chnl. Blkr. | | Calcium Channel Blocker |
| Norvasc® | Calc. Chnl. Blkr. | | Calcium Channel Blocker |
| Atorvastatin | Cholesterol | | Statin |
| Crestor® | Cholesterol | | Statin |
| Ezetimibe | Cholesterol | | Cholesterol absorption inhibitors |
| Fenofibrate | Cholesterol | | Fibric Acid Derivatives |
| Gemfibrozil | Cholesterol | | Fibric Acid Derivatives |
| Lipitor® | Cholesterol | | Statin |
| Lopid® | Cholesterol | | Fibric Acid Derivatives |
| Lovastatin | Cholesterol | | Statin |
| Mevacor® | Cholesterol | | Statin |
| Pravachol® | Cholesterol | | Statin |
| Pravastatin | Cholesterol | | Statin |
| Rosuvastatin | Cholesterol | | Statin |
| Simvastatin | Cholesterol | | Statin |
| Tricor® | Cholesterol | | Fibric Acid Derivatives |
| Vytorin® | Cholesterol | | Statin |
| Zetia® | Cholesterol | | Cholesterol absorption inhibitors |
| Zocor® | Cholesterol | | Statin |
| Carvedilol | Congestive Heart Failure | Hypertension | Beta Blocker |
| Coreg® | Congestive Heart Failure | Hypertension | Beta Blocker |
| Digoxin | Congestive Heart Failure | Atrial Fibrillation | Anti-Arrhythmic |
| Lanoxin® | Congestive Heart Failure | Atrial Fibrillation | Anti-Arrhythmic |
| Spiriva® | COPD | | Bronchodilator |
| Tiotropium | COPD | | Bronchodilator |
| Benzonatate | Cough | | Antitussives |
| Tessalon® | Cough | | Antitussives |
| Aricept® | Dementia | | Cholinesterase inhibitors |
| Donepezil | Dementia | | Cholinesterase inhibitors |
| Exelon® | Dementia | | Cholinesterase Inhibitors |
| Rivastigmine | Dementia | | Cholinesterase Inhibitors |
| Amitriptyline | Depression | | Anti-depressant |
| Celexa® | Depression | | Anti-depressant |
| Citalopram | Depression | | Anti-depressant |
| Cymbalta® | Depression | | Anti-depressant |
| Desvenlafaxine | Depression | | Anti-depressant |
| Desyrel® | Depression | | Anti-depressant |
| Duloxetine | Depression | | Anti-depressant |
| Effexor® | Depression | | Anti-depressant |
| Elavil® | Depression | | Anti-depressant |
| Escitalopram | Depression | | Anti-depressant |
| Fluoxetine | Depression | | Anti-depressant |
| Lexapro® | Depression | | Anti-depressant |
| Mirtazepine | Depression | | Anti-depressant |
| Nortriptyline | Depression | | Anti-depressant |
| Pamelor® | Depression | | Anti-depressant |
| Paroxetine | Depression | | Anti-depressant |
| Paxil® | Depression | | Anti-depressant |
| Pristiq® | Depression | | Anti-depressant |
| Prozac® | Depression | | Anti-depressant |
| Remeron® | Depression | | Anti-depressant |
| Sertraline | Depression | | Anti-depressant |

## Common Medications and Conditions Treated

| Drug | Primary Condition Treated | Other Conditions Treated | Drug Class |
|---|---|---|---|
| Trazodone | Depression | | Anti-depressant |
| Venlafaxine | Depression | | Anti-depressant |
| Zoloft® | Depression | | Anti-depressant |
| Actos® | Diabetes | | Oral Diabetic |
| Diabeta® | Diabetes | | Oral Diabetic |
| Glyburide | Diabetes | | Oral Diabetic |
| Januvia® | Diabetes | | Oral Diabetic |
| Pioglitazone | Diabetes | | Oral Diabetic |
| Sitagliptin | Diabetes | | Oral Diabetic |
| Levemir® | Diabetes | | Insulin |
| Lantus® | Diabetes | | Insulin |
| Novolog® | Diabetes | | Insulin |
| Humalog® | Diabetes | | Insulin |
| Amaryl® | Diabetes | | Anti-Diabetic |
| Glimepiride | Diabetes | | Anti-Diabetic |
| Glucophage® | Diabetes | | Anti-Diabetic |
| Liraglutide | Diabetes | | Anti-Diabetic |
| Metformin | Diabetes | | Anti-Diabetic |
| Onglyza® | Diabetes | | Anti-Diabetic |
| Saxagliptin | Diabetes | | Anti-Diabetic |
| Victoza® | Diabetes | | Anti-Diabetic |
| Glipizide | Diabetes(II) | | Oral Diabetic |
| Glucotrol® | Diabetes(II) | | Oral Diabetic |
| Enoxaparin | DVT | PE | Anti-coagulant |
| Lovenox® | DVT | PE | Anti-coagulant |
| Pradaxa® | DVT | PE | Anti-coagulant |
| Oseltamivir | Flu | | Anti-Viral |
| Tamiflu® | Flu | | Anti-Viral |
| Diflucan® | Fungal Infections | | Anti-Fungal |
| Fluconazole | Fungal Infections | | Anti-Fungal |
| Ketoconazole | Fungal Infections | | Anti-Fungal |
| Nizoral® | Fungal Infections | | Anti-Fungal |
| Esomeprazole | GERD | | Proton Pump Inhibitors |
| Omeprazole | GERD | | Proton Pump Inhibitors |
| Pantoprazole | GERD | | Proton Pump Inhibitors |
| Dexlansoprazole | GERD | | Proton Pump Inhibitors |
| Ranitidine | GERD | | H2 Antagonists |
| Famotidine | GERD | | H2 Antagonists |
| Metoclopramide | GERD | | GI Stimulants |
| Rabeprazole | GERD | | Proton Pump Inhibitors |
| Lansoprazole | GERD | | Proton Pump Inhibitors |
| Nexium® | GERD | | Proton Pump Inhibitors |
| Prilosec® | GERD | | Proton Pump Inhibitors |
| Protonix® | GERD | | Proton Pump Inhibitors |
| Dexilant® | GERD | | Proton Pump Inhibitors |
| Zantac® | GERD | | H2 Antagonists |
| Pepcid® | GERD | | H2 Antagonists |
| Reglan® | GERD | | GI Stimulants |
| Aciphex® | GERD | | Proton Pump Inhibitors |
| Prevacid® | GERD | | Proton Pump Inhibitors |
| Allopurinol | Gout | Kidney Stones | Anti-Gout |
| Zyloprim® | Gout | Kidney Stones | Anti-Gout |
| Ticagrelor | Heart Disease | | Anti-Platelet |
| Brilinta® | Heart Disease | | Anti-Platelet |
| Avapro® | Hypertension | | Angiotensin Receptor Blockers |
| Diovan® | Hypertension | | Angiotensin Receptor Blockers |
| Irbesartan | Hypertension | | Angiotensin Receptor Blockers |
| Valsartan | Hypertension | | Angiotensin Receptor Blockers |
| Enalapril | Hypertension | | ACE Inhibitor |

## Common Medications and Conditions Treated

| Drug | Primary Condition Treated | Other Conditions Treated | Drug Class |
|---|---|---|---|
| Lisinopril | Hypertension | | ACE Inhibitor |
| Prinivil® | Hypertension | | ACE Inhibitor |
| Vasotec® | Hypertension | CHF | ACE Inhibitor |
| Accupril® | Hypertension | | ACE Inhibitor |
| Benazepril | Hypertension | | ACE Inhibitor |
| Lotensin® | Hypertension | | ACE Inhibitor |
| Quinapril | Hypertension | | ACE Inhibitor |
| Atenolol | Hypertension | Angina | Beta Blocker |
| Bystolic® | Hypertension | | Beta Blocker |
| Lopressor® | Hypertension | | Beta Blocker |
| Metoprolol | Hypertension | Angina | Beta Blocker |
| Nebivolol | Hypertension | | Beta Blocker |
| Tenormin® | Hypertension | Angina | Beta Blocker |
| Clonidine | Hypertension | | Anti-Adrenergic |
| Diltiazem | Hypertension | | Calcium Channel Blocker |
| Losartan | Hypertension | | Angiotensin Receptor Blockers |
| Ramipril | Hypertension | | Angiotensin Converting Enzyme Inhibitors |
| Hydralazine | Hypertension | | Vasodilators |
| Propranolol | Hypertension | | Beta Blocker |
| Hyzaar® | Hypertension | | Angiotensin Inhibitors |
| Catapres® | Hypertension | | Anti-Adrenergic |
| Cardizem® | Hypertension | | Calcium Channel Blocker |
| Cozaar® | Hypertension | | Angiotensin Receptor Blockers |
| Altace® | Hypertension | | ACE Inhibitor |
| Apresoline® | Hypertension | | Vasodilators |
| Inderal® | Hypertension | | Beta Blocker |
| Levothyroxine | Hypothyroidism | | Thyroid Drugs |
| Synthroid® | Hypothyroidism | | Thyroid Drugs |
| Oxybutynin | Incontinence | | Urinary Antispasmodics |
| Ditropan® | Incontinence | | Urinary Antispasmodics |
| Amoxicillin | Infection | | Antibiotic |
| Amoxil® | Infection | | Antibiotic |
| Azithromycin | Infection | | Antibiotic |
| Biaxin® | Infection | | Antibiotic |
| Cefdinir | Infection | | Antibiotic |
| Ceftin® | Infection | | Antibiotic |
| Cefuroxime | Infection | | Antibiotic |
| Cephalexin | Infection | | Antibiotic |
| Cipro® | Infection | | Antibiotic |
| Ciprofloxacin | Infection | | Antibiotic |
| Clarithromycin | Infection | | Antibiotic |
| Cleocin® | Infection | | Antibiotic |
| Clindamycin | Infection | | Antibiotic |
| Flagyl® | Infection | | Antibiotic |
| Keflex® | Infection | | Antibiotic |
| Levaquin® | Infection | | Antibiotic |
| Levofloxacin | Infection | | Antibiotic |
| Macrobid® | Infection | | Antibiotic |
| Metronidazole | Infection | | Antibiotic |
| Minocin® | Infection | | Antibiotic |
| Minocycline | Infection | | Antibiotic |
| Nitrofurantoin | Infection | | Antibiotic |
| Omnicef® | Infection | | Antibiotic |
| Pen VK® | Infection | | Antibiotic |
| Penicillin | Infection | | Antibiotic |
| Zithromax® | Infection | | Antibiotic |
| Adalimumab | Inflammatory Conditions | | Anti-Inflammatory |
| Deltasone® | Inflammatory Conditions | | Anti-Inflammatory |
| Humira® | Inflammatory Conditions | | Anti-Inflammatory |

## Common Medications and Conditions Treated

| Drug | Primary Condition Treated | Other Conditions Treated | Drug Class |
|---|---|---|---|
| Omnipred® | Inflammatory Conditions | | Anti-Inflammatory |
| Prednisolone | Inflammatory Conditions | | Anti-Inflammatory |
| Prednisone | Inflammatory Conditions | | Anti-Inflammatory |
| Ibuprofen | Inflammatory Conditions | Pain | NSAID |
| Celecoxib | Inflammatory Conditions | Pain | NSAID |
| Naproxen | Inflammatory Conditions | Pain | NSAID |
| Advil® | Inflammatory Conditions | Pain | NSAID |
| Celebrex® | Inflammatory Conditions | Pain | NSAID |
| Aleve® | Inflammatory Conditions | Pain | NSAID |
| Meloxicam | Inflammatory Conditions | Pain | NSAID |
| Mobic® | Inflammatory Conditions | Pain | NSAID |
| Diclofenac | Inflammatory Conditions | | NSAID |
| Voltaren® | Inflammatory Conditions | | NSAID |
| Zolpidem | Insomnia | | Sedative |
| Ambien® | Insomnia | | Sedative |
| Sumatriptan | Migraine | | Anti-Migraine |
| Imitrex® | Migraine | | Anti-Migraine |
| Dramamine® | Nausea | | Antiemetic |
| Meclizine | Nausea | | Antiemetic |
| Ondansetron | Nausea | | Antiemetic |
| Zofran® | Nausea | | Antiemetic |
| Risedronate | Osteoporosis | | Bisphosphonates |
| Alendronate | Osteoporosis | | Bisphosphonates |
| Raloxifene | Osteoporosis | | Selective Estrogen Receptor Modulators |
| Actonel® | Osteoporosis | | Bisphosphonates |
| Fosamax® | Osteoporosis | | Bisphosphonates |
| Evista® | Osteoporosis | | Selective Estrogen Receptor Modulators |
| Hydrocodone | Pain | | Narcotic Analgesics |
| Tramadol | Pain | | Narcotic Analgesics |
| Oxycodone | Pain | | Narcotic Analgesics |
| Codeine | Pain | | Narcotic Analgesics |
| Vicodin® | Pain | | Narcotic Analgesics |
| Ultram® | Pain | | Narcotic Analgesics |
| Percocet® | Pain | | Narcotic Analgesics |
| OxyContin® | Pain | | Narcotic Analgesics |
| Tylenol® #2 | Pain | | Narcotic Analgesics |
| Etanercept | Rheumatoid Arthritis | | TNF Alfa Inhibitors/Antirheumatics |
| Enbrel® | Rheumatoid Arthritis | | TNF Alfa Inhibitors/Antirheumatics |
| Abilify® | Schizophrenia | Bipolar Depression | Anti-Psychotic |
| Aripiprazole | Schizophrenia | Bipolar Depression | Anti-Psychotic |
| Latuda® | Schizophrenia | | Anti-Psychotic |
| Lurasidone | Schizophrenia | | Anti-Psychotic |
| Olanzapine | Schizophrenia | Bipolar Depression | Anti-Psychotic |
| Quetiapine | Schizophrenia | | Anti-Psychotic |
| Risperdal® | Schizophrenia | | Anti-Psychotic |
| Risperidone | Schizophrenia | | Anti-Psychotic |
| Seroquel® | Schizophrenia | Bipolar Depression | Anti-Psychotic |
| Zyprexa® | Schizophrenia | Bipolar Depression | Anti-Psychotic |
| Dilantin® | Seizures | | Anti-Convulsant |
| Lyrica® | Seizures | | Anti-Convulsant |
| Phenytoin | Seizures | | Anti-Convulsant |
| Pregabalin | Seizures | | Anti-Convulsant |
| Depakote® | Seizures | | Antiepileptic |
| Divalproex | Seizures | | Antiepileptic |
| Gabapentin | Seizures | | Antiepileptic |
| Lamictal® | Seizures | | Antiepileptic |
| Lamotrigine | Seizures | | Antiepileptic |
| Neurontin® | Seizures | | Antiepileptic |
| Topamax® | Seizures | | Antiepileptic |

| Drug | Primary Condition Treated | Other Conditions Treated | Drug Class |
|---|---|---|---|
| Topiramate | Seizures | | Antiepileptic |
| Keppra® | Seizures | | Anti-Seizure |
| Levetiracetam | Seizures | | Anti-Seizure |
| Bactroban® | Staph Infection | | Topical Antibiotic |
| Mupirocin | Staph Infection | | Topical Antibiotic |

# COMMON HCC CODING QUESTIONS/ISSUES

If the documentation states the patient has chronic kidney disease (CKD) stage III, and the provider has ordered an ultrasound of the kidney and bladder for elevated creatinine, should I code the elevated creatinine or CKD as the reason for the ultrasound on an outpatient encounter?

As per Coding Clinic, Q2, 2013, since elevated creatinine levels are expected in CKD, you would code 585.3-CKD III, as the reason for the ultrasound, with the elevated creatinine code listed second.

There is no change in the rationale of this answer due to ICD-10 implementation. See section N18 for CKD.

Are diagnoses documented on interpreted diagnostic reports found in the medical record acceptable for risk adjustment? (i.e. cardiology and vascular surgeons, interventional radiology, neurology and pulmonology

No. They have to be incorporated in the physician's progress notes. These services alone are not acceptable for risk adjustment. The service must be a face to face service by an appropriate physician type, not a test result.

If a hospitalist evaluates a patient in the hospital do we follow inpatient or outpatient coding guidelines? Can we submit this data to the health plan?

Yes, submit the hospitalist's data to the health plan. Follow the physician/outpatient coding guidelines (Coding Clinic 2000 Q3). All physician services should be submitted to the health plan and the plan submits them to CMS.

Yes, a hospitalist's services may be submitted, using the Outpatient Coding Guidelines. There is no impact due to ICD-10 implementation.

If the MD writes under one DOS: Assessment : 1) COPD 2) ASTHMA. Then the following visit he/she writes just COPD, do you capture only the COPD, or code ICD-9: 493.21 (Chronic obstructive asthma with status asthmaticus) on the first date of service, and don't code the COPD alone for the second visit?

In coding, each chart note stands alone. You don't look back at earlier chart notes to determine how the current one should be coded. You cannot use diagnoses documented at an earlier encounter to supplement the diagnosis in the current encounter. It also seems that you're assuming that if the physician writes:

COPD
Asthma

That the patient has chronic obstructive asthma with status asthmaticus. That's not the case. Status asthmaticus is a life threatening condition, characterized by intractable wheezing (e.g. an asthma attack) that does not respond to the usual treatment of bronchodilators and steroids. In order to code 493.21, the physician must state that the patient has chronic obstructive asthma with status asthmaticus, not COPD and asthma.

The correct coding, if both COPD and asthma are documented on the same date, is 493.20 - Chronic obstructive asthma, unspecified. This is because the coding notes for this section of the ICD-9 indicate the following :

"Asthma with chronic obstructive pulmonary disease [COPD]".

You would not code 496, COPD, because the coding notes for 496 indicate: "Note: This code is not to be used with any code from categories 491-493"

Under ICD-10, the diagnostic statement "COPD" is coded J44.9 Chronic obstructive pulmonary disease, unspecified. However, there is a note in this section which instructs coders to also code the type of asthma, if present. Asthma codes are found in section J45.

### Can we code from the chief complaint

No, the CC is the patient's explanation of what is wrong with them. The patient is not qualified to make a diagnosis.

### How are pathologic (compression) fractures of the vertebrae coded?

Pathologic fractures of the vertebrae are coded 733.13. Although the Official Coding Guidelines indicate that the condition should not be coded on an ongoing basis, a recent Coding Clinic (Q3 2008) indicates that if the patient is being treated for a non-healing pathologic fracture, it can be coded as often as treated.

Please refer to Chapter 13 c. of the Official Guidelines for Coding and Reporting of ICD-10 codes for instructions on coding Pathologic Fractures.

### Do you continue to report AAA even after it has been surgically repaired?

No. Per the coding guidelines, you do not code conditions that no longer exist. From the Official ICD-9 Coding Guidelines:

Section IV. Diagnostic Coding and Reporting Guidelines for Outpatient Services

K. Code all documented conditions that coexist
Code all documented conditions that coexist at the time of the encounter/visit, and require or affect patient care treatment or management. Do not code conditions that were

previously treated and no longer exist. However, history codes (V10-V19) may be used as secondary codes if the historical condition or family history has an impact on current care or influences treatment.

There is no change in the rationale for this answer due to ICD-10 implementation. The same instruction appears in Section IV J in ICD-10.

Recently, we received advice that we may amend our medical records to reflect lab data or other new information weeks after the service is rendered. The advice also said that we could then submit corrected diagnosis data for risk adjustment without another face-to-face visit. Is this correct? A. There is no change in the rationale for this answer due to ICD-10 implementation.

CMS allows physicians to create an addendum to medical records to reflect confirmation of a diagnosis under certain circumstances. However, the example given by CMS is several days, not weeks, after a visit. Most laboratory and radiology services have results within days, not weeks, and it is expected that addenda will be completed as soon as possible after receipt of the additional information. CMS published this guidance in a training guide that has been removed from the CSSC website, and is no longer available. However, it reads as follows:

### 6.4.2 Unconfirmed Diagnoses

Physicians and hospital outpatient departments shall not code diagnoses documented as "probable," "suspected," "questionable," "rule out," or "working." Rather, the condition(s) shall be coded to the highest degree of certainty known for that encounter/visit, such as symptoms, signs, abnormal test results, or other reason for the visit. CMS recognizes that this is an area where the physician-reported diagnosis and hospital inpatient diagnosis for the same encounter may disagree since hospital inpatient rules allow for coding of suspected conditions as if they were confirmed.

It also is understood that the physician record is not a static document. Positive test results and notation regarding contact with the patient for a revised plan of treatment often are added to the record several days after the patient encounter. When these addenda are made, corrections or additions to the diagnoses submitted to the MA organization may be recommended especially if the HCC assignment is impacted.

### Example: 4

A physician removes a mole during an office visit and sends the specimen for pathology. The diagnoses documented are "suspicious skin lesion" (709.9, not in model) and "rule out melanoma." At this point, the diagnosis 709.9 may be submitted, but the diagnosis of melanoma may not. The pathology report is returned several days later and confirms malignant melanoma. The physician reviews the findings, initials the report, and documents in the record the results and notification to the patient. Since the removal of the mole was done during the office visit, the new code (172.9, melanoma) should be submitted with that date of service.

There is no change in the rationale for this answer due to ICD-10 implementation. The ICD-10 guidelines are consistent.

My question concerns the signature requirements for MA RADV. Is a signature log acceptable or only a signature attestation? I have heard both are acceptable but would like to clarify. Thank you.

For an MA RADV a Signature Attestation is the only acceptable form of signature verification. As it stands, Signature Logs are used for Fee for Service only. When CMS conducts a RADV audit, they will provide official signature attestations.

There is no change in the rationale of this answer due to ICD-10 implementation.

In a review of a medical record there is a statement, "please see the attached record, administered today". If the attached record is available to the coder at the time of this medical record review, can it be used as supporting documentation for that DOS, using outpatient guidelines?

It depends what it is—if it's something that this physician did **and interpreted**, like an EKG you can use it. If it's something another physician did, most often, the physician must agree with what was said in their notes.

There is no change in the rationale of this answer due to ICD-10 implementation.

What is the correct code for inferior infarct, age undetermined?

It appears that you are referring to the computerized analysis of an EKG. A physician MUST interpret the EKG in order for any coding to take place. A. Under ICD-10, physicians will need to be more specific, classifying myocardial infarctions as either STEMI or NSTEMI in order for them to be coded.

Below are the facts that I gathered that might help you to guide me in order to utilize the acute renal failure. Acute Renal Failure (584.9) has a model category 135 with a risk factor of 0.476 based on 65-69 year old patient. CKD 4, 5, and ESRD (585.4, 585.5, 585.6) has a model category 136 and 137 respectively with a risk factor of 0.224 based on 65-69 years old patient. CKD 4, 5, and ESRD superseded by Acute Renal Failure due to higher risk factor. Unspecified CKD (585.9), Nephropathy (583.81), CKD 1, 2, 3 (585.1, 585.2, 585.3) are no longer risk adjusting for 2014. Is that appropriate to use acute renal failure due to DM or Hypertension in physician based coding? Is it appropriate to use acute renal failure instead of CKD 1, 2, or 3 in physician based coding?

To answer your questions, it is never appropriate to code anything except what the physician has documented in the medical record. If the physician has documented acute renal failure for a patient with diabetes then it is appropriate to code it. If the physician notes that the patient has CKD (chronic kidney disease) a coder or anyone responsible for coding, can never change that diagnosis to acute renal failure in order to code based on what pays the most. You must code what is documented in the medical record. The Official ICD-9 Coding Guidelines should always be your guide, no matter what type of chart review you are performing. Coding for conditions that are not documented in the medical record is considered fraud. I recommend you review both the AAPC code of ethics at: http://www.aapc.com/AboutUs/code-of-ethics.aspx and the AHIMA code of ethics: here. Finally, all coding must be supported by what is documented in the medical record for each date of service and conform to-The Official ICD-9 Coding Guidelines, which can be downloaded at: http://www.cdc.gov/nchs/data/icd/icd9cm_guidelines_2011.pdf

There is no change in the rationale of this answer due to ICD-10 implementation. You can download the current ICD-10 guidelines at http://www.cdc.gov/nchs/icd/icd10cm.htm


What is the correct code for Coronary Artery Disease (CAD)?

The correct code for coronary artery disease depends on what information is provided in the documentation. CAD is commonly miscoded as 414.00 (coronary atherosclerosis of unspecified type of vessel, native or graft). However, this is incorrect unless the physician specifically notes that both native and graft vessels are present. Hence, the documentation must include information regarding a previous coronary artery bypass graft (CABG) in order to use this code. When there is no documentation of a prior CABG, then the correct code for CAD is 414.01, coronary atherosclerosis of native coronary artery even though the physician does not state "native artery." This rule was published in Coding Clinic For ICD-9 CM 2nd quarter, 1995 and reiterated in 1st quarter, 2004.

Under ICD 10, the correct code for Coronary Artery Disease is I25.10 Atherosclerotic heart disease of native coronary artery without angina pectoris.


My query is whether CMS will accept the Diagnosis codes reported from the superbills. In a chart provider has documented the assessment of a patient in the superbill instead of progress notes. For e.g., There is a patient record with the DOS 01/29/09 for which both superbill & progress notes is available. Progress note has Chief Complaint, Vital Signs, ROS & Objective. The assessment was given in the superbill at the bottom.

No, CMS specifically says that superbills are not a part of the medical record. See the 2008 Risk Adjustment Data Technical Assistance Participant Guide, page 170. Superbills can only be used to collect data, not as a part of the medical record.

There is no change in the rationale for this answer due to the implementation of ICD-10.

A hospice patient had a face-to-face encounter with their PCP and chronic diseases were documented in the medical record. Do we get paid using the Risk Adjustment model for patients enrolled in hospice?

No, hospice enrollees are not paid using the Risk Adjustment method.

Please see pgs 23-24 in the CMS Managed Care Manual, which can be downloaded from the from the [CMS website](#), regarding payment for hospice enrollees.

Also, payment lags 1 year behind the service in the risk adjustment model, and you don't receive payment for a patient who expires. The nature of hospice (a physician certifies that the patient has less than 6 months to live) means that most patients won't be alive in the payment year. A patient must be a member in the payment year in order for the group to receive payment.

There is no change in this answer due to ICD-10 implementation.


**If the Provider's Assessment and Plan states the following, is it ok to assume that the DM and the Manifestation below are linked because they are listed under the same number/bullet in the A&P? 1. DM, Retinopathy 2.HT**

Yes, this is generally considered to be supportive of the linkage between the two. However, there is no linkage documented if they are on separate bullet points.


**Can I code h/o CVA, left sided weakness due to CVA with 438.20? I know in the ICD-9 coding books it states, Hemiplegia/hemiparesis, when I look up the definition of hemiparesis in the medical dictionary, it states: "Weakness on one side of the body, less severe than hemiplegia". So wouldn't the appropriate code be 438.20 since the meaning of hemiparesis is one sided weakness?**

The correct code assignment, according to the Coding Clinic Q1, 2005, for CVA late effects stated as weakness, code- 438.89 (Other late effects of CVA) and 728.87 (Muscle weakness) The documentation must state Hemiplegia or Hemiparesis in order to use the 438.2X series.

There is a new Coding Clinic (Q1 2015) that indicates that residual R(L) sided weakness following a CVA is to be coded as hemiplegia. The codes for hemiplegia following a CVA are I69.251-I69.259.


**If it's documented in the record, that the patient has a history of alcoholism, and has been without alcohol for 1 year now, how should I code this?**

As per Coding Clinic the correct way to code is from the Alcohol Dependence Syndrome category 303, with the 5th digit of "3" to indicate that the patient is in remission. This is very commonly not coded correctly.

There is no change in the rationale of this answer due to ICD-10 implementation.
F10.21 Alcohol dependence, in remission


If you have documentation of ESRD due to type 1 diabetes and HTN would you add v45.11 for dialysis if it is not mentioned?

No. Only documented conditions can be coded. You cannot assume the patient is receiving dialysis—they may have chosen not to do so.

There is no change in the rationale of this answer due to ICD-10 implementation.


A PCP had a face-to-face visit with a patient on 11/16/07, but on 12/19/07 he added a note for "chart review" and 2 diagnoses that were previously not documented in the patient's medical record. Would it be acceptable to report these 2 additional diagnoses to CMS? One of the diagnoses added does risk adjust.

No, it is not acceptable to report the 2 additional diagnoses from the "chart review." Coding from "chart reviews," "failed visits," or any other progress notes that are not from a face-to-face visit with a patient are not valid sources for risk adjustment coding. This guideline is in the 2008 Risk Adjustment Data Technical Assistance Participant Guide in section 3.2.4.

There is no change in the rationale for this answer due to ICD-10 implementation.


Once a patient has had a kidney transplant is it correct to still code CKD?

It is correct to code CKD if it still exists, and is documented. A transplanted kidney can leave a patient with CKD, but again, the physician must document that CKD exists in order to capture it. You would never assume that the patient has CKD under any circumstances.

There is no change in the rationale for this answer due to ICD10 implementation.


When reviewing records, if we find "depression" documented three times or more in a twelve-month period, can we assign code 296.30 for major depression, recurrent episode?

Under the Official ICD-9 Coding Guidelines, a diagnosis can only be coded when it is explicitly spelled out in the medical record. It cannot be inferred (even when a provider does the coding) that depression documented multiple times in a record is "major recurrent depression." Also, the Diagnostic Coding and Reporting Guidelines for Outpatient Services, pgs 88-91, explain that a diagnosis is often not established during the first visit and it may take subsequent visits to confirm that diagnosis. All diagnoses should be supported by physician documentation.

The physician should clearly document the type of depression in order to assign a more specific diagnosis code such as major depressive disorder. If only depression is documented, code 311 "depression not otherwise specified."

Official ICD-9 Coding Guidelines can be downloaded on the CDC website.

There is no code for "depression, not otherwise specified" under ICD-10, which crosswalks to major depressive disorder. It is critical that physicians document the type of depression that the patient has in order to ensure the best code selection possible.


How do I code a CVA?

If the only documentation is "CVA" the default code is 434.91 (CVA –stroke, ischemic). However, if the physician specifies the type of stroke (embolic, hemorrhagic, etc) there are separate codes in the 434.XX section of the ICD-9.

However, these codes are for use during the acute event—i.e., while the patient is still hospitalized. Once the patient has been discharged from the hospital, then coding and documentation should indicate a history of stroke (V12.54). More importantly, sequelae, what ICD-9 calls "late effects" should be documented and coded. Late effects such as hemiplegia/hemiparesis secondary to CVA (438.2X), aphasia (438.11) should be documented and coded. (Coding Clinic, Q4 2004)

Without further documentation, the best code would be I63.9.


Patient was seen for follow up surgery for "Left knee status post hardware removal for tibial plateau fracture, currently with pes bursitis" and they received an injection. Do I code a Follow up V67.09 along with 726.61 Pes Anserine Bursitis- 20610-RT and injection- J1040 / 80 mg Depo Medrol or would I not code the follow-up code? Also, this is out of the global period.

Even though out of the global, if the physician states a surgery f/u, I would bill all four codes as listed. Depending on the insurance, you may not be paid separately for the Depo Medrol.

Under ICD-10 this would be coded Z09 Encounter for follow-up examination after completed treatment for conditions other than malignant neoplasm and M76.899 Other specified enthesopathies of unspecified lower limb, excluding foot.


What is the criteria for Chronic (Non – Viral) Hepatitis i.e. ICD 9 code 571.40?

Coding Clinic, 1993 Q4, indicates that this code is used when there is a diagnostic statement of "active chronic hepatitis". The indication that it is active seems to be important, since most hepatitis caused by medications often resolves when the medication is stopped. When possible, the physician should be queried for more information if the only statement is "chronic hepatitis" since the cause of the hepatitis (medications, alcohol, viral) is important in correct code assignment.

The ICD10 code K73.9 Chronic hepatitis, unspecified does not seem to have any specific Coding Clinic instructions at this time.

I have a question. If a providers documents diagnoses of COPD, but the ICD9 code submitted is 491.0 (simple chronic bronchitis). Is this correct coding?

No, the physician cannot choose a code more specific than his/her documentation. If the documentation indicates "COPD" it is incorrect coding to call it simple chronic bronchitis when he/she chooses a code. The correct code for a diagnosis of COPD is 496.

There is no change in the rationale for this answer under ICD-10. The coder (or physician) can never choose a code more specific than the documentation

Many providers want to continue to perform Annual Wellness Visits and evaluate and treat all of their stable chronic conditions at the same time. The code the CPT code for the preventative exam then add a modifier 25 and add 99213 or 99214. According to ICD-10, Z00.00 Encounter for general examination w/o complaint or abnormal findings. This has an Excludes1 note: encounter for examination of signs and symptoms – code to sign or symptom. Z00.01 Encounter for general adult medical exam with abnormal findings. Is this appropriate?

There's no change in CMS' policy regarding a wellness visit and a chronic condition management condition on the same day. You would NEVER attach a code that says the patient has no signs and symptoms to the chronic care visit. That's what diagnosis code pointers are for. The patient's actual diagnoses should be submitted, not Z00.00.

One of our providers asked, " What do I document if a patient had atrial fibrillation in the hospital but was cardioverted and doesn't have it anymore? Does the patient still have atrial fibrillation?"

What is unclear is whether or not the patient remains on treatment with medication. If the patient is being treated with medication to control their atrial fibrillation going forward, then the atrial fibrillation is under control, not "cured", and it would be appropriate to continue to report it. If the patient is not on ongoing treatment, then the health plan and medical group are entitled only to one year reimbursement (generated by the hospital's submission) of

Atrial fibrillation, because the patient no longer has (and is no longer being treated for) atrial fibrillation.

There is no change in the rationale for this answer under ICD-10.

I am doing chart review for HCC Risk Adjustment, I have a chart where the physician put down "Recurrent DVT of RLE, chronic" and they have assigned code 451.2 next to it in the A/P. I would like to code it 453.50 for risk adjustment, is this possible, or do you have to go with the code in the chart and then educate the physician?

Coding is never based on what is payable, but always based upon the narrative documentation that the clinician has provided. This physician has not stated that the patient has chronic DVT, only that it has recurred—it could be the 1st recurrence, or the 100th—the documentation does not state. It's unclear what the word "chronic" refers to. You can't assume that because it's recurrent it's chronic; they simply are not the same thing. However, there is nothing that says you must use the same code the physician does, especially when it does not match the documentation they have provided. In this case, the physician has described a DVT—which is appropriately coded 453.40 per ICD-9. If you are in a situation where you can query the physician for clarification (within a few days of the service) this would be a great situation to do that. If not, I would not code the "chronic" wording. You may want to use this as an educational example with the physician.

There is no change in the rationale of this answer due to ICD-10 implementation. The coder may choose a different code than the physician has chosen. I suggest you educate the physician about your code choice.

## What are the ICD-10 codes for the following diseases/symptoms
7 KB

Headache and dizziness R51, R42, chest pain and palpitation R07.9, R00.2, exertional dyspnea R06.09, slowing of speech, R47.89, generalized weakness, M62.81, Benign prostatic hyperplasia N40.0

If the patient is a diabetic, and the note indicates that the patient has retinopathy, do you assume it's diabetic retinopathy?

ICD-9 does not generally assume a cause and effect relationship between diabetes and other illnesses. Because the physician did not state a causal relationship, through terms like "diabetic retinopathy", or "retinopathy secondary to diabetes", or "diabetes with retinopathy", the correct coding is 362.10, background retinopathy NOS and, if the note indicates that the patient is diabetic, 250.00, DM II, not stated to be uncontrolled. This is a change from the longstanding Coding Clinic advice that the physician must state the causal relationship.

The ICD-10 also does not generally assume a causal relationship. Unspecified background retinopathy is coded H35.00-Unspecified background retinopathy. DM II without complications is coded E11.9-Type 2 diabetes mellitus without complications.

### Can angina still be coded and reported for a patient that is status post stenting?

It's appropriate to report angina post stenting only if the patient still has angina. If the stent resulted in resolution of the patient's angina, it should not be reported.

There is no change in the rationale for this answer due to the implementation of ICD-10.

### If the patient has both diabetes and peripheral neuropathy, how should this be coded?

If the documentation indicates only diabetes and peripheral neuropathy, then the documentation is 250.00 (uncomplicated type II diabetes) and 357.2 diabetic polyneuropathy. Unless the physician specifically states that the polyneuropathy is a complication of the diabetes, or documents "diabetes with polyneuropathy", then the two diseases are considered unrelated. This is a change from the longstanding Coding Clinic advice that the physician must state the causal relationship.

The ICD-10 still requires a causal relationship be stated. If it is stated, the correct code is E11.40 Type 2 diabetes mellitus with diabetic neuropathy, unspecified.

### In order to improve a patient's RAF score, do all of the patient's diagnoses need to be documented on their wellness visit and progress notes each time they are seen by a physician? In other words, do the progress notes require documentation of all diagnoses for each visit?

The purpose of a Wellness Visit is to get an overall picture of the patient's health, and healthcare needs. Other visits may be done for a number of reasons---but under no circumstances should any visit—wellness or otherwise, be performed simply to "collect" diagnoses. Because of the purpose of an Annual Wellness Visit (i.e., getting a snapshot of the patient's overall health, and implementing care where needed), it does provide a good opportunity to **assess** any of a patient's conditions---particularly chronic conditions. Other visits are usually performed as needed to assess and treat specific conditions, **based upon a patient's needs**. In either case, where conditions are assessed and/or treated, it is appropriate at that time to document not only the diagnosis, but any treatment, response to treatment, etc.

If your question is "how often must a diagnosis be reported in order for it to be risk adjusted in the next year, each diagnosis must be captured at least once per year. However, any time a physician or other clinician assesses or implements treatment for a condition, it should be documented and submitted, not only for risk adjustment purposes, but to provide a complete and accurate picture of the patient's health.

There is no change in the rationale of this answer due to ICD-10 implementation.


**The physician has noted that the patient has a pacemaker, CHF, and CAD. For risk adjustment coding, do we code all three? My understanding is that if patient has a working pacemaker then we drop all cardiac related codes.**

Not all cardiac conditions require a pacemaker. While CHF often requires a pacemaker, a non-specific diagnosis like CAD would not. According to Coding Clinic, 1993, 5th issue, if the patient with CHF and a pacemaker still requires ongoing medication for their CHF, then the CHF should be coded.

There is no change to the rationale of this answer due to ICD-10 implementation.


**If the patient has DM, dyslipidemia and HTN can I link the HTN to DM, using 250.80 DM II with specific manifestations?**

No. You cannot assume an association between the two conditions. Remember, these codes represent conditions caused by diabetes, not merely co-existing with diabetes. This causal relationship must be stated specifically by the physician. For example "hyper/dyslipidemia due to diabetes and/or HTN 2° to diabetes. Many patients have these conditions long before they were diagnosed with diabetes, so 250.80 would not be appropriate.

There is no change to the rationale of this answer due to ICD-10 implementation.


**If there is a report in the patient's chart and you cannot identify the physician or provider name, is it acceptable to code from this report for risk adjustment?**

No, you cannot code a diagnosis if you cannot determine who the rendering the provider is. CMS will only accept diagnoses from complete documentation, which must have the diagnosis documented, as well as have the patient's name, date of service, a unique patient identifier (e.g. date of birth or medical record number) and be performed and legibly signed by an acceptable rendering provider (e.g., physician, physician extender, inpatient hospital, or outpatient hospital).

There is no impact due to ICD-10 implementation.

**If the patient has both diabetes and peripheral vascular disease, how should this be coded?**

If the documentation indicates only diabetes and peripheral vascular disease, then the documentation is 250.00 (uncomplicated type II diabetes) and 443.9 Peripheral vascular disease, unspecified. Unless the physician specifically states that the peripheral vascular disease is a complication of the diabetes, or the physician notes "diabetes with peripheral vascular disease" or similar wording, then the two diseases are considered unrelated. This is a change from the longstanding Coding Clinic advice that the physician must state the causal relationship.

Under ICD-10 this is coded E11.59-Type 2 diabetes mellitus with other circulatory complications.


**Are hospitalists considered an acceptable physician specialty for risk adjustment purposes? If so what code is used for data collection? EX – General Practice is code 01.**

Hospitalist isn't a true specialty, rather an explanation of where the physician works. Most hospitalists are internal medicine physicians, although a few are of various other specialties. In order to tell if the physician is an acceptable physician specialty you'll need to look further, perhaps contacting the physician for his/her board certification. Note that neither providers or health plans actually submit the physician specialty codes to CMS at this time.

There is no change in the rationale for this answer due to the implementation of ICD-10.


**Our endocrinologist is documenting Diabetes Mellitus type 1.5. I queried him about what should be coded, DM I or DM II, since there is no ICD-9 code for DM 1.5. He stated it should be coded as DM I, since the patient does not have an autoimmune component to their diabetes and is not type II. Is this the correct way to code DM type1.5?**

At this time, there is no ICD-9 code for Diabetes Mellitus Type 1.5. As per Coding Clinic, Q3, 2013, if you are able to query the provider to determine if type I or type II DM is correct. Otherwise, DM II is the default for unspecified Diabetes Mellitus code with 250.00.

There is no change in the rationale of this answer due to ICD-10 implementation. See E11.9 for type 2 diabetes mellitus without complications.


**Can CAD be related to Diabetes? What would be the codes?**

From a coding perspective, CAD can be "related to" or caused by or secondary to diabetes only if the physician says so in their documentation. This is why we strongly recommend that physicians be trained in documentation. It doesn't matter if the physician thinks that the diabetes caused the CAD if they don't say so. The coder cannot make that assumption.

If the physician documents CAD secondary to the diabetes, then the correct coding would be 414.01 (see earlier question in "Ask a Coder") and 250.8X – diabetes with other specified manifestations.

The correct code is E11.59-Type 2 diabetes mellitus with other circulatory complications.

Can you please verify the accurate codes for s/p craniotomy with residual left sided paralysis and aphasia dx (344.32, 784.3 or 438.22, 438.11) It is unknown if the patient is suffering from brain lesions or traumatic brain injury?

The correct codes for hemiparesis (one-sided paralysis) are in 342.9X- Hemiplegia, unspecified section, not in the section for the sequelae for stroke, since this is unrelated to a stroke. 784.3 is correct for aphasia not related to a stroke.

The codes for hemiplegia are found in section G81Hemiplegia and hemiparesis, and R47.01 for Aphasia.

I continuously have a doctor that puts 'same' in the diagnosis field of the EMR or he will put "same as x-ray findings" Is this allowable? If not, PLEASE help me to explain to him that it's not.

There is no diagnosis code for "same"—I think that's the best information you can give the physician. Diagnosis coding (or procedural coding for that matter) is always based upon the narrative documentation on this date of service. The physician must provide a narrative diagnosis on this date of service, in order for coding to be done. The physician is placing you and your organization at risk in the event of an audit. I suggest that you enlist the assistance of your manager or better yet, your organizations physician champion to counsel this physician about proper documentation.

There is no change in the rationale of this answer due to ICD-10 implementation.

What is the correct code for a follow up visit to a physician's office for a patient who has had a myocardial infarction that is less than 8 weeks old? 410.90 or 410.92. Please advise.

There isn't quite enough information to precisely answer the question, but I'll give you enough information so you can determine what the correct 5th digit is. I assume by the way your question is phrased that the physician did not state the area of the heart muscle affected by the MI, which led you to the fourth digit of "9".

Generally, for a patient being seen in the office it won't ever be a fifth digit of 1.

First, the diagnosis code will always be determined by the documentation in the physician record.

The fifth-digit of "0" (unspecified episode of care) means the physician did not provide enough information to determine what episode of care the patient is in.

The fifth-digit of "1" (initial episode of care) covers all care provided to a newly diagnosed myocardial infarction patient until the patient is discharged from medical care (i.e., discharged from the hospital). This includes any transfers to and from other facilities prior to the patient's discharge and occurring within the eight-week time frame.

The fifth-digit of "2" (subsequent episode of care) covers care (further observation, evaluation or treatment) rendered after the initial treatment (discharge), but the myocardial infarction is still less than 8 weeks old.

Once the MI is more than 8 weeks old, the physician should document old MI (ICD-9-CM 412)

Under ICD-10, an Acute MIs are found under STEMI and NSTEMI in the ICD10 (I21) and they are only coded for the first 4 weeks. After that, the code for old MI (I25.1) should be used.


It is true that under the ICD10 coding guidelines we can code a r/o (rule out) diagnosis that if were exist? For example: The doctor writes : r/o Diabetes Mellitus type II

No, there is no change in the coding of rule out or suspected diagnoses. A physician may only code confirmed diagnoses.


I have question regarding Past Medical History. Can coder capture from Past Medical History if member still on treatment?   Does provider need to diagnoses it in Assessment

CMS has indicated in their 2008 RAPS Participant Guide that a "history of" diagnosis raises confusion whether or not a disease is current. Because medications can be used for so many illnesses, being "on treatment" for a disease is really for the doctor to determine, not the coder. The best course of action is to query the physician (if the patient was seen within the past few days) or educate the physician. This way, records going forward will be clear and not prevent coding problems.


If a patient has type II diabetes, do we need to also code V58.67 if the patient is on insulin? We are coding 250.00 for diabetes, but don't want to upcode or overcode. Is adding V58.67 deemed to be upcoding or overcoding and will we run into compliance issues? Will adding this code lead to an extra risk score?

No, it is not upcoding or overcoding for two reasons:

1. The Coding Clinic calls the use of V58.67 optional ("if desired") (Coding Clinic 2004 Q4)
2. It doesn't lead to a higher or extra risk score. Both V58.67 and 250.00 or 250.01 group to HCC 19. You don't get paid for HCC 19 twice no matter how many times that you

submit the code during the collection period.

There is no reason not to code all applicable diagnoses, since they give CMS a more complete picture of our members. Many diagnoses not in the Risk Adjustment model are part of the RxHCC (Part D) model, so it is important to code all diagnoses, not just diagnoses that lead to an HCC.

The correct code for Long term use of Insulin is Z79.4. As with ICD-9, use of this code does not trigger an "extra" HCC, and may be coded if documented by the physician.


My question is, if the patient has pacemaker implant for SSS or complete AV block, would you code SSS or AV block in addition to V45.01 for Pacemaker status?

According to Coding Clinic, 1993, issue 5, not usually:

Although it can be argued that sick sinus syndrome (SSS) is an ongoing condition controlled by a pacemaker, no code assignment is required if no attention or treatment is provided to the condition or device. This differs from the ongoing medication administration provided for conditions such as congestive heart failure, hypertension or diabetes mellitus, and therefore, justifying code assignment. The use of V45.0, Cardiac pacemaker in situ is optional; some facilities will want to code the presence of the device for tracking purposes. Use of code V45 .0 does not imply management of the pacemaker, only its presence.

So, if no treatment is rendered specific to the arrhythmia or the device, no coding should take place. If there is treatment directed at the arrhythmia, then the pacemaker likely is not performing as it should be. If the pacemaker requires reprogramming, then it would be appropriate to code the SSS.

There is no change in the rationale of this answer due to ICD10 implementation.


The physician has documented "aplastic anemia/ vit B12 deficiency. Recent hemoglobin and hematocrit of 10/29.5 and WBC of 7". While the patient's hemoglobin and hematocrit values have been consistently low over the course of a couple of years, all of her other CBC vales are within normal limits. A previous record from the same physician reads "acquired anticoagulation factor deficiency and pernicious anemia". There is no documentation of more serious bone marrow disorders in any note. Should the physician be queried to provide more supporting documentation regarding his choice of diagnosis of aplastic anemia? Reference I have read state that pancytopenia can be caused by B 12 deficiency. Would that (284.1) be a better choice?

Unless the visit was within the past few days, it's too late to query the physician. I don't believe that coding aplastic anemia under these circumstances would be appropriate. It appears that the physician may be thinking "aplastic anemia vs. (/) vitamin B12 deficiency" (pernicious anemia, 281.0). But it doesn't seem like the physician has made a solid diagnosis.

Aplastic anemia can only be confirmed by bone marrow biopsy, and there isn't one of those. That doesn't mean that one hasn't been done, but the statements are too unclear. Although we can't code from those earlier diagnostic statements, they do serve to demonstrate that there is some confusion over the actual diagnosis.

We can't make choices like this---nor can the doctor. If he's documented pernicious anemia, but the patient really has pancytopenia, then he cannot choose pancytopenia just because he knows that's what it is...he needs to make an amendment with the correct diagnosis (within a few days) or make a correct and complete diagnosis at the next visit.

I recommend that you educate him/her regarding the documentation issues in this case, and ask for a clear diagnostic statement at the patient's next visit.

There is no change in the rationale of this answer due to ICD10 implementation.


I have several questions about Morbid Obesity, and am hoping you can help me:
- If the physician documents morbid obesity but the BMI is not documented, can we code?
    - Per Coding Clinic, Q3 2011, if there is no conflicting information, the morbid obesity can be coded without a BMI noted.
- If the BMI is documented but morbid obesity is not documented, can we code morbid obesity?
    - No. Per Coding Clinic, Q3 2011, the physician must document the significance of the BMI. If he makes no comment on it, then morbid obesity may not be coded.
- If the physician documents obesity and the BMI is 42, can we code morbid obesity?
    - No. Per the Official Guidelines for Coding and Reporting, you cannot code this, because the information is conflicting. If the documentation is recent (under 72 hours) you may query the physician for an updated diagnosis. Remember, queries cannot be leading.
- If BMI is 38 and Dr. Documents as morbid obesity, can we code morbid obesity?
    - No. Per the Official Guidelines for Coding and Reporting, you cannot code this, because the information is conflicting. If the documentation is recent (under 72 hours) you may query the physician for an updated diagnosis. Remember, queries cannot be leading.

There is no change to the rationale of this answer due to ICD-10 implementation.


If the patient has type 2 diabetes with the following complications due to the diabetes; Peripheral neuropathy, Peripheral vascular disease, Cataracts, Insulin use. Would the correct codes be: 250.60, 357.2, 250.70, 443.81, 250.50 and 366.41? Is it correct coding to code 3 different diabetes codes?

Yes, you can code as many diabetes codes as apply. Because this patient has Type 2 diabetes and is on insulin, you should also add V58.62, long term use of insulin.

Because the diabetes codes are now combined with the specific complication, the correct codes would be: E11.36 Type 2 diabetes mellitus with diabetic cataract; E11.40 Type 2 diabetes mellitus with diabetic neuropathy, unspecified; E11.59 Type 2 diabetes mellitus with other circulatory complications; Z79.4 long term (current) use of insulin.

What documentation would we look for to support the codes 303.90 (other and unspecified alcohol dependence, unspecified drunkeness) and 303.91 (other and unspecified alcohol dependence, continuous drunkenness)? Dr. is documenting ETOH ½ pint Vodka everyday OR ETOH abuse. What info will validate these codes if this will not?

In the case of "ETOH ½ pint Vodka everyday", nothing can be coded. A coder can't make any diagnosis, and the doctor has just stated how much the patient drinks. He/she hasn't said that there's abuse OR dependence (the codes you are asking about are dependence (i.e., addiction) codes). In order to code addiction/dependence, the physician must document that the patient is addicted or dependent on alcohol. In order to use the fifth digit of "1" the physician must indicate that continuous drunkenness is present.

In the case of the statement "ETOH abuse", then you can only code 305.00, Nondependent alcohol abuse, unspecified drunkenness. The physician has stated that abuse (not dependence) is present. The physician has not specified continuous or episodic drunkenness, so only the unspecified fifth digit of "0" is appropriate.

There is no change in the rationale for this answer due to ICD-10 implementation. The codes for alcohol abuse are found in F10.xx of the ICD-10.

If the provider only documents "DM with renal manifestations" and no mention of the 'type' of manifestation, can the 250.40 and 583.81 still be coded?

No. In that case, you cannot code 583.81—diabetic nephropathy. We can never assume what a problem is. Not all renal complications of diabetes are nephropathy. If you look at the instruction 250.4 you see:

Use additional code to identify manifestation, as:
chronic kidney disease (585.1-585.9)
diabetic:
nephropathy NOS (583.81)
nephrosis (581.81)
intercapillary glomerulosclerosis (581.81)
Kimmelstiel-Wilson syndrome (581.81)

From this, it's clear that more than one renal complication—and this is not an all inclusive list. The physician must document what the complication is. If he doesn't the only thing that can be coded is the diabetes.

There is no change in the rationale for this answer under ICD-10. The codes for diabetes with kidney complications are found under E11.2x-Type 2 diabetes mellitus with kidney complications.

Will a coder consider carpal tunnel syndrome as a peripheral neuropathy? That is, would they code both carpal tunnel syndrome and peripheral neuropathy?

No. A coder would never choose to extrapolate from carpal tunnel syndrome, which has its own code (354.0) to a peripheral neuropathy, many of which have their own codes. If a condition has its own code, only that code that should be used. The only exception would be if there is a coding instruction that instructs otherwise.

The codes for peripheral neuropathies include a description and/or diagnosis that informs the coder (and physician) what types of conditions they represent. As you can see, these are quite different from a condition like carpal tunnel syndrome.

356.0 Hereditary peripheral neuropathy
Déjérine-Sottas disease

356.1 Peroneal muscular atrophy
Charcot-Marie-Tooth disease, etc.

There is no change in the rationale for this answer due to ICD-10 implementation. When there is a specific code for a condition, only that code is to be used. Section G56.0 Carpal tunnel syndrome is to be used for carpal tunnel syndrome.

Scenario 1: Patient came with HA, dizziness. Vitals: BP 145/90 (for example). PMH - HTN, CKD. Final diagnosis - Hypertension alone. Is it appropriate to code 403.xx, 585.x (My argument - Once 403.xx, 585.x was assigned on a patient's medical record, It should be coded as 403.xx, 585.x on the forthcoming visits (even-though if the physician final impression noted HTN alone) due to chronic nature of HTN and CKD or 403.xx, 585.x can be coded only if CKD in final impression? Scenario 2: Patient came with HA, dizziness. PMH - No HTN. BP: 145/90 (for example). Final impression: Hypertension. Is it appropriate to code 401.9 or 796.2 (Transient hypertension). My argument - Still, a coder cannot assume and code a diagnosis. If, 796.2 is your answer (because HTN not in PMH) means, at what stage we can come to know that, really patient with HTN or just transient HTN in order to code appropriately?

Scenario 1: I believe you can only code exactly what is documented ON THAT DAY. You never assume anything based on a prior diagnosis. Let me give you a good reason why. In between visits, the patient has a kidney transplant, and no longer has CKD. If you've assumed CKD just because the patient had it in the past, you've now coded something that no longer exists and should not be coded.

Scenario 2: As you said, coders cannot assume. Unless the physician states that the patient has transient hypertension, then hypertension is coded as 401.9---because that's what the doctor documented. If he/she meant transient hypertension, then he/she would say so. I personally do not code from the PMH in physicians' charts—the Coding Clinic that talks about coding chronic conditions is clearly directed at hospitals, and I would rather be safe than sorry.

There is no change in the rationale of this answer due to ICD-10 implementation.

The physician mentions DM2 onset date 4.30.15. Throughout the note he is not addressing DM anywhere except the problem list. Can we code DM2 based on problem list alone

No, CMS has clearly said in old User Group documents (see page 3 of the Feb. 2008 User Group Q and A) that you cannot code from unconfirmed problem lists

If I'm coding for my physician seeing hospitalized patients, do I use the Inpatient Coding Guidelines?

No. The Inpatient Coding Guidelines are for use by the facility only. Physicians use the Outpatient guidelines, no matter what the place of service is. This is supported by Coding Clinic, 4th Quarter, 2000, which states in part: "When coding for physician services, whether provided in the hospital inpatient setting or in the physician office, coders should be guided by the Diagnostic Coding and Reporting Guidelines for Outpatient Services (Hospital- Based and Physician Office). The inpatient guidelines are for hospital coding".

No. Per Coding Clinic, Q 1 2014, the Outpatient Guidelines are to be used for all physician services, irrespective of place of service. This is also stated in the Section IV. Diagnostic Coding and Reporting Guidelines for Outpatient Services of the Official Guidelines for Reporting ICD-10.

If a NP or PA is submitting claims, will they receive a Risk Score? Since they do not have members assigned to them, but to the PCP, will they receive a RA score or does it go to the supervising provider's score?

Providers do not have risk scores. Certain of our reports show the risk average risk score of the members assigned to a PCP, or members seen by a given specialty, but these are always a reflection of the members' risk scores.

Most physician extenders are not individually credentialed by health plans. IF they are identified as the rendering provider on incoming encounters (something that doesn't happen consistently) it might be possible to determine the average risk score of members seen by the physician extender. But, it would not be a unique score, since there would always be overlap with the PCP that the members are assigned to.

There is no change in the rationale for this answer due to the implementation of ICD-10.


"Carotid stenosis and arterial vascular disease, no complicating CVA" is documented. Can we code 433.10 and 440.9 or do we need to code 447.9? What would be the correct code. Can you please clarify this?

The correct code for carotid stenosis without a CVA is 433.10. Coding "arterial vascular disease" is not possible—the physician has not stated WHERE it is. Is it peripheral? Is it in the carotid? Is it in the coronary arteries? As a coder, you cannot make a diagnosis. When the physician is unclear, you cannot code.

There is no change in the rationale of this answer due to ICD-10 implementation. The code range for carotid stenosis is I65.21-I65.29, depending on documentation. As noted before, arterial vascular disease in this context is vague and should be clarified with the physician.


What if the patient develops complications from tracheostomy scars - like difficulty or pain when swallowing, voice impairment-- because of these ongoing issues can the tracheostomy status code be coded year over year? The physician is reviewing these issues with the patient and documenting in the visit notes.

You cannot code for tracheostomy status when the tracheostomy is closed. Tracheostomy status means the patient has a functioning stoma, or opening into the trachea.

If there are complications from an actual tracheostomy, there are codes in the 519.0 series for complications of a tracheostomy. Use of these codes is limited to when the physician documents that a complication of a tracheostomy is present.

There is no change in the rationale for this answer due to the implementation of ICD-10. Tracheostomy complications are found in J95.x of the ICD-10.


The documentation states CKD only, with no stages assigned, and in the progress note under plan it states, "Patient on chronic dialysis, will continue with current dialysis treatment" How should I code this?

As per Coding Clinic, Q2, 2013, when the documentation states Chronic kidney disease and the patient is on chronic dialysis as well, you may use code 585.6. This is an exception to the rule that nothing is assumed in coding. Also, code V45.11 for Renal dialysis status. However, if the documentation states chronic kidney disease with acute kidney failure on dialysis, you would code acute kidney failure- 584.9 and chronic kidney disease- 585.9 along with V45.11. Only code 585.6 if documentation states on "chronic" dialysis. Rationale: Patients can also receive dialysis treatment for an episode of acute kidney failure and only be in stage II or III CKD.

There is no change in the rationale of this answer due to ICD-10 implementation. See section N18 for CKD.

If a physician documents "Chronic Diastolic Heart Failure" and "Congestive Heart Failure" and does not link them, would they need to address each separately or is it an assumed relationship?

No, there are very few assumed relationships in ICD-9 or ICD-10. Both diagnoses should be coded separately.

There is no change in the rationale of this answer due to ICD-10 implementation. Note that under ICD-10, systolic heart failure is automatically noted to be CHF.

If a person has LAD stenosis, but it was stented, do we still code the stenosis?

The Official Coding Guidelines address this situation.

K. Code all documented conditions that coexist
Code all documented conditions that coexist at the time of the encounter/visit, and require or affect patient care treatment or management. Do not code conditions that were previously treated and no longer exist. However, history codes (V10-V19) may be used as secondary codes if the historical condition or family history has an impact on current care or influences treatment."

The purpose of a stent is to ensure that the vessel is patent and that the stenosis no longer exists. If the stenosis no longer exists, it should not be coded.

This same instruction can be found in Section IV J of the ICD-10 Official Guidelines for Coding and Reporting

I would like to know some opinions regarding to coding the following documentation by Physician: " Vascular Dementia". In my opinion I'll use 290.40 plus 437.0. Please see instructional notes " Use additional code to identify cerebral atherosclerosis". I need your opinion.

You only use an additional code if the condition documented. It's not something that is automatically done, or done based on what you know about disease processes. Based on your email, the physician only documented vascular dementia. If the physician had said vascular dementia due to cerebral atherosclerosis, then you would code it.

The instructional notes for 250.40 say: Use additional code, to identify manifestation, as:

chronic kidney disease (585.1-585.9)
diabetic:
nephropathy NOS (583.81)
nephrosis (581.81)
intercapillary glomerulosclerosis (581.81)
Kimmelstiel-Wilson syndrome (581.81)

But you don't code any of those things unless they are documented. Vascular dementia NOS is indexed to 290.40. In this case, the vascular dementia is not otherwise specified, and you would not assume or code cerebral atherosclerosis.

There is no change in the rationale of this answer due to ICD10 implementation. Vascular dementia without behavioral disturbance is coded F01.50 in ICD-10.


A person came into the ER with a bleeding laceration and was taped up, went home and back to the hospital 2 days later for additional bleeding. What is the dx for the 2nd admission? Patient also had acute blood loss anemia.

If the physician documented acute blood loss anemia in regard to this laceration that should be the principal diagnosis, followed by the laceration, which hasn't yet healed.

There is no change in the rationale of this answer due to ICD-10 implementation


I am looking for some clarification on how I would code "History of osteomyelitis at 9 yrs of age with residual shortening of the leg" (This pt is 67 yrs old). Would 730.18 (chronic osteomyelitis) +731.3 (major osseous defects) be appropriate?

The physician clearly indicated that there is a history of osteomyelitis. It's unlikely that the patient would still have a bone infection 58 years later. The correct coding would be 736.81, acquired unequal leg length, and V13.59, personal history of other musculoskeletal disorders.


If a physician documents "weakness" in the physical exam for extremities, is that considered enough support for a diagnosis of history of CVA with left hemiparesis for CMS Risk Adjustment?

Unless the physician states that the patient has hemiparesis due to/secondary to the CVA, it cannot be coded. CMS Risk Adjustment follows all coding rules and guidelines, including those in Coding Clinic. This issue was addressed in Q1 2005, and the question asked if weakness secondary to a CVA should be coded as hemiparesis secondary to CV A. CC advised that the correct coding of weakness secondary to CVA is 438.89 (other late effects of cerebrovascular disease) and 728.87, muscle weakness. Physicians should be educated about the need for clear documentation for ICD-9 coding purposes. This is one of the scenarios I use in training, since it's so commonplace.

A new Coding Clinic for ICD-10 indicates that R or L sided weakness due to CVA is coded as I69.35x, Hemiplegia and hemiparesis following cerebral infarction, a change from previous guidance.

My understanding of CMS' new criteria for signatures is that as of January 1, 2009, CMS will not accept a stamped signature on a progress note. The provider's name must be spelled out with their credentials on each page. Does this do away with the provider signature logs?

Signature logs are not the same as a signature stamp. A signature stamp replaces a physical signature. As of 1-1-09, CMS does not accept signature stamps under any circumstances.

CMS has said (on a RADV conference call) that they will not accept signature logs. Although signature logs are acceptable in fee-for-service Medicare, as of this time, CMS will not accept them for Medicare Advantage patients.

There is no change in the rationale for this answer due to the implementation of ICD-10.

What are the codes for ASHD due to HTN. Do you consider this a hypertensive heart disease 402.90 or just 414.01, 401.9? Please advise. Thanks

I would not code 402.90 unless the physician clearly says hypertensive heart disease or something similar. ASHD is a disease of the vessels leading to the heart, and it is usually caused by HTN, smoking or hypercholesterolemia. The correct coding is 414.01 and 401.9.

There is no change in the rationale of this answer due to ICD-10 implementation. The correct coding is I70.90 Unspecified atherosclerosis and I10 Essential (primary) hypertension.

What diagnosis code should you use if a physician documents "CKD, stage 3-4" I thought that if I was able to find information that stated if a physician documents this that you should code to the higher level of CKD, but I cannot find that information now. Any advice?

I would not use the higher—it's critical that in an audit, the diagnosis be supported. It's unlikely that there will be support for the higher level present on the date of service.

There is no change in the rationale of this answer due to ICD-10 implementation

If the physician states dilated aorta or slightly dilated aorta at 4 cm, would it be appropriate code an aneurysm?

No. Coders can only code what is documented. The physician may feel that this dilation is clinically insignificant, and does not constitute an aneurysm.

There is no change to the rationale of this answer due to ICD-10 implementation.

The physician documented: "Intra-Aortic Calcification. Chronic, clinically stable. Recommended statin today. Pt will think about it more and let me know. c/w baby aspirin." Does this documentation justify coding 440.0 (atherosclerosis of the aorta)?

You have to look at the medical record (the date of service) as a whole in order to know if something can be coded. If this is all of each record, I wouldn't code them. If this is just the assessment (i.e., the diagnosis), and there is documentation to support each diagnosis, then they could be coded—except probably the first one. "Abnormal GFR" doesn't mean anything. If a normal GFR is 90-120 then an 89 is "abnormal", but it doesn't mean the patient is sick. The physician has to not only write diagnoses, but they have to have support and they have to make sense.

There is no change in the rationale of this answer due to ICD10 implementation. Atherosclerosis of the aorta is coded I70.0 Atherosclerosis of aorta in ICD10.


We have a new member, she is in for her H&P. She was hit by a car last November, suffered multiple traumatic injuries supracondylar femur fracture, fractures of the 9th & 10th ribs with pneumothorax, scalp laceration. How do I code this?

It's hard to determine what the patient is being seen for. All of the conditions listed could only be coded as a "history of" IF they were assessed. What should be coded is what the patient was seen and assessed for today. None of these things listed seem to be current conditions.

Risk Adjustment never changes what it is appropriate to code. What we have to be mindful of is what physicians (especially) have often forgotten to code—current conditions that they assess, but don't mark on a superbill; and what physicians have often forgotten to DOCUMENT, so that they can be reminded to do so. For example physicians often have assessed long term chronic problems (like the labs on an A fib patient, or the cardiac status and evaluation for peripheral edema in a CHF patient) but have forgotten to write the diagnosis for these conditions. Education focused on documentation is critical so that physicians are accurately recording what they assess.

There is no change in the rationale for this answer due to ICD-10 implementation.

What is the diagnosis code for uncontrolled hypertension?

The ICD-9 does not categorize hypertension by level of control. Hypertension is categorized as benign or malignant. If a note indicates only "uncontrolled hypertension", the correct coding is 401.9, "hypertension, unspecified". If there is hypertensive heart or kidney disease present, these should be noted and coded in the 402.X or 403.X range. You should not code 401.1 unless your documentation says that the hypertension is benign.

The ICD-10 does not categorize hypertension by level of control. Further, ICD-10 no longer categorizes hypertension as benign or malignant. If the documentation indicates only "uncontrolled hypertension", the correct ICD-10 code is I10, essential hypertension.


I need some help regarding sequelae from CVA. A provider assessed disturbances of visions due to an old CVA I went to the late effect sections on ICD-10 book, when I got to that section, it pointed me out to see also sequelae I69.90-Unspecified sequelae of unspecified cerebrovascular disease. On that same list, there was a phrase in red that says "use additional code to identify the sequelae". My question is – isn't it the disturbance of vision is already the sequelae"? So what other additional code should I add? Please advise.

No, the visual disturbance isn't included in I69.90, which is described as Unspecified sequelae of unspecified cerebrovascular disease- that could be any one of multiple "unspecified sequelae", so it doesn't tell someone running reports, or doing epidemiological studies (some of the primary reasons for coding besides billing and payment) what the problem is. Since there is limited information in the documentation, the best code to use is probably: H53.10 Unspecified subjective visual disturbances. This code tells someone what kind of sequela it is. This will be necessary many times when you use an unspecified code, because they can be so many things.


Would the code V12.51 be used for history of DVT?

Yes. You should also use V58.61 if long term use of anti-coagulants is documented.

The correct ICD-10 codes are Z86.718 Personal history of other venous thrombosis and embolism and Z79.01 Long term (current) use of anticoagulants.


Can you explain the difference between late effects and after care for fractures? I am in orthopedics and have had two different pieces of advice about fracture care and late effects. Any help you could give would be appreciated.

The coding guidelines for late effects and acute fractures vs. aftercare of fractures is below. The Official Coding Guidelines can be downloaded at: http://www.cdc.gov/nchs/datawh/ftpserv/ftpicd9/ftpicd9.htm#guidelines.

**Acute Fractures vs. Aftercare**

Traumatic fractures are coded using the acute fracture codes (800-829) while the patient is receiving active treatment for the fracture. Examples of active treatment are: surgical treatment, emergency department encounter, and evaluation and treatment by a new physician.

Fractures are coded using the aftercare codes (subcategories V54.0, V54.1, V54.8, or V54.9) for encounters after the patient has completed active treatment of the fracture and is receiving routine care for the fracture during the healing or recovery phase.

Examples of fracture aftercare are: cast change or removal, removal of external or internal fixation device, medication adjustment, and follow up visits following fracture treatment.

Care for complications of surgical treatment for fracture repairs during the healing or recovery phase should be coded with the appropriate complication codes.

Care of complications of fractures, such as malunion and nonunion, should be reported with the appropriate codes.

Pathologic fractures are not coded in the 800-829 range, but instead are assigned to subcategory 733.1X.

There is no change in the rationale for this answer. Aftercare codes for injuries are found in the Z section of ICD-10.


I am hoping I can ask you a coding question regarding diabetes. If a physician bills 250.60 and the manifestation is NOT billed does/can that code stand alone or does it get downcoded to 250.00 by CMS? Also, if the physician coded 250.60, with no second code selected and manifestation not clearly identified, how can we rebill with the manifestation?

In the first scenario, no, CMS doesn't downcode it. It is just processed as submitted. Of course, it must be documented in the medical record appropriately.

In the second scenario, again, CMS does not change the code, but would not allow it in a Risk Adjustment Data Validation. If you identify that the physician didn't document a complication, then you should submit an adjustment transaction to SCAN with 250.00, diabetes without complications.

Under ICD-10, all diabetes codes for complications include the specific complication (and not a group of complications) so this problem cannot occur.

**What is the correct code for neuropathy found in a podiatry chart?**

The ICD-9 indexes the term "neuropathy" to 355.9. The physician's specialty or type of provider does not influence coding, since one can't infer anything when coding. Even though a podiatrist most likely means polyneuropathy, we can't use that knowledge to choose a code. 355.9 is neuropathy NOS and is the correct code if any provider documents "neuropathy."

There is no index term for "neuropathy" in ICD-10, meaning physicians will have to be more specific with their documentation


**Good morning, If a patient has chronic kidney disease and is hospitalized for acute renal failure, can we (as the provider not facility) code for both conditions 585.9 and 584.9?**

What a provider can code is always driven by two things:

- What the provider documented
- What the ICD-9 coding rules allow

The provider cannot code for any condition he did not document himself, irrespective of what the patient was hospitalized for.

There is no coding rule which says that these are mutually exclusive conditions. If your provider's documentation supports both conditions, then both can be coded.

A. There is no change in the rationale for this answer due to the implementation of ICD-10. Both N17.9 Acute kidney failure, unspecified and N18.9 Chronic kidney disease, unspecified can be billed.

There is no change in the rationale for this answer due to the implementation of ICD-10. Both N17.9 Acute kidney failure, unspecified and N18.9 Chronic kidney disease, unspecified can be billed.

---

**If additive RAF points are added for disease interactions: "CHF_COPD" = 0.259, etc. Does the interaction count only when the actual diagnosis of CHF 428.0 is used, or any diagnosis in the same HCC as CHF, such as diastolic heart failure? Does the interaction count only when the actual diagnosis of COPD 496 is used, or any diagnosis in the same HCC as COPD, such as chronic bronchitis?**

The interaction codes are applied when any diagnosis code in the same HCC is coded.

Made in the USA
Columbia, SC
22 March 2019